KABOOM!

*The Method Used By Top Dentists
for Explosive Marketing Results*

By Wendy O'Donovan Phillips

ISBN: 150314397X
ISBN 13: 9781503143975
Library of Congress Control Number: 2014920311
CreateSpace Independent Publishing Platform
North Charleston, South Carolina

To all of the dentists
for all of the care you have given.

And to Mom
for completing the painting.

TABLE OF CONTENTS

INTRODUCTION   vii
   From Mystery to Method   vii
   How to Use This Book   xi
PART ONE: THE FOUNDATION OF THE *KABOOM!*
METHOD   1
   Survey the Patients and Team   3
   Construct a Marketing Message and Design   9
   Build a Balanced Marketing Formula   15
   Top 10 Common Mistakes in Setting the Foundation 29
PART TWO: BRAND AWARENESS   31
   The Science Behind the Logo   33
   Adding a Tagline   39
   A Technique for Signs   41
   Top 10 Common Mistakes in Brand Awareness   43
PART THREE: TRADITIONAL MEDIA   45
   Direct Mail Debunked   47
   Print Advertising Strategy   53
   Blueprint for Billboard Advertising   61
   Foolproof Broadcast Advertising   63
   Top 10 Common Mistakes in Traditional Media   67
PART FOUR: ONLINE PROMOTION   71
   Disciplined Website Design   73
   Demystifying Social Media   79
   A System for Attracting Web Visitors   85

Reputation Management Simplified   95
Top 10 Mistakes in Online Promotion   99
PART FIVE: INTERNAL MARKETING   101
Checklist for Team Training   105
Referral Mining on LinkedIn   109
Referral System   113
The Trifecta   117
Top 10 Mistakes in Internal Marketing   123
AFTERWORD   125
Exercise #1: Your Message and Design Equation   127
Exercise #2: Your Balanced Marketing Formula   129
Sample Balanced Marketing Formula   131
STAY ON THE CUTTING EDGE   133
ACKNOWLEDGEMENTS   135

FROM MYSTERY TO METHOD

Dr. Brett Kessler had been enjoying private practice for several years when he suddenly found himself overwhelmed with competitors encroaching on his market. Seven dentists had opened within a mile of his office. He felt confused about how to stand apart from them, and his original marketing strategies weren't doing the trick.

Quietly, his patients leaked away to some of the surrounding dental practices. His production dwindled. He knew he was great at what he did and no one was quite like him, yet his patients couldn't recall why they should be loyal to him.

It took a toll on him personally as well as professionally. He was nationally known for his dental approach, yet he was feeling down and out.

Dr. Kessler is not alone. Dentists everywhere are increasingly boggled by marketing.

Social media marketing is all the rage these days – why not try a little of that? The Yellow Pages ad worked for decades – why doesn't it anymore? Referrals occasionally come to the practice – but how to get more? The practice never had to market before – hopefully patients will still come...

Hope is not a method. There is an actual methodology to marketing:

1. Survey the patients and team
2. Define a Message and Design Equation
3. Build a Balanced Marketing Formula, or 12-month marketing plan
4. Deploy the plan for steadfast results!

This is the *KABOOM!* method. This is the method that I used with Dr. Kessler. I worked with him to understand his vision for his practice and his production goals. We put into writing a baseline of where he was at that moment and where he wanted to be in 12 months. I asked him about his best patients, those who accepted his advice and followed treatment plans. They turned out to be his strongest stories of transformation. I surveyed those patients with a questionnaire to find out what they appreciated about his work. In the process, they revealed how they went about finding him and what other dentists they considered. Then I looked closely at his competitors to see what they were delivering. I shared what I learned with Dr. Kessler.

From the verbatim survey responses, we were able to define exactly the message that resonated most with patients, and therefore their peers – or potential new patients. We articulated that message in writing. We also put to paper what design best matched that message. Together, these two things became Dr. Kessler's Message and Design Equation. This tool helped us stay consistent in how the practice's marketing spoke, looked and felt.

Then it came time to construct a Balanced Marketing Formula, or marketing plan. Based again upon the survey results, Dr. Kessler and I collaborated on how best to tell the unique story about his practice, and differentiate his from the others within a mile, and well beyond. We set out to invite his perfect patient population to his door. We agreed to do just four tactics in his Balanced Marketing Formula:

1. Create an upscale *logo* to best represent his brand
2. Refresh his *website* with improved messaging to attract his ideal patients
3. Launch a robust *print advertising* campaign to attract even more patients
4. Ratchet up his program of word-of-mouth *referrals* to create patient loyalty and yet more new patients

That's it. Just the four. These were the vehicles, or tactics, to get him re-energized. His unique formula for success. And we had the data to back it.

Over the months that followed we put the Balanced Marketing Formula to work.

And it worked!

Dr. Kessler was more interested in quality than quantity. He didn't want huge new patient volume; rather, he wanted to attract a small number of just the right patients that would get the most out of his unique approach.

The *KABOOM!* method helped Dr. Kessler do just that.

The *KABOOM!* method has helped countless more dentists enjoy validation of their marketing efforts, higher returns on marketing investments, more stability in patient traffic and production dollars, steady growth and increased practice value.

The *KABOOM!* method is based upon research and work with hundreds of dental practices over the years. Practices like Dr. Kessler's. Practices like yours.

HOW TO USE THIS BOOK

There are three ways to get the most out of this book, independent of each other or mixed together:

1. **Do-It-Yourself Guide.** If you want total control and prefer to create the marketing, do the *KABOOM!* method yourself. Follow the step-by-step instructions for everything needed to do to be successful, with occasional help from outsiders.
2. **Marketing Handbook.** Perhaps a staff member handles your marketing, with input and approvals from you. In that case, work together on the exercises at the end of the book to lay the foundation for the *KABOOM!* method. Once that is in place, leave the creation and delivery of the marketing to him or her, using the method as a guide.
3. **Litmus Test.** Maybe you prefer to outsource the marketing to an agency and focus the team exclusively on patient care. If that's the case, use the *KABOOM!* method to test whether the agency's solutions really work. The detailed approach of these lessons will help hold them accountable.

PART ONE

THE FOUNDATION OF THE *KABOOM!* METHOD

The method starts with surveying the patients and team, defining a Message and Design Equation, and building a Balanced Marketing Formula as a 12-month marketing plan. Once this foundation is set, you will be well equipped to launch your marketing, tactic by tactic. Part One shows how to set the foundation, and Parts Two, Three, Four and Five detail how to launch each marketing tactic. Let's begin.

Survey the Patients and Team

The first step is to ask the happiest patients the right questions to understand how they think about the practice and how they consume marketing. An emailed survey looks simple to the patient, yet it provides immense insight into the practice. This section will lay out how to effectively survey patients.

Why survey? When you survey patients, you get timely, relevant and actionable feedback. You learn precisely what they love most about the practice, and it's typically not the things that come to mind first. It's not technology. It's not philosophy. It's not even credentials. The thing they love best is that *you made life better*.

When surveyed correctly, patients light up and share animated stories. Only the patients have the passion behind the story, and that shines through when they start talking about you. You couldn't make this stuff up if you tried.

Here's how Dr. Kessler talks about what he does best: "I am a dentist specializing in comprehensive dental care for patients with a focus on TMJ disorder treatment, and I have been in practice more than 20 years."

By contrast, here is how I, as one of his happy patients, talk about what he does best: "When I came to see Dr. Kessler, I was getting migraine headaches and missing work left and right. Life was all about managing pain. In a matter of a few visits, Dr. Kessler totally restored me back to my happy self. I'm more productive at work than ever before. And I am even able to go running again, which I haven't been able to do in months."

Doctors tend to talk about features rather than benefits. Happy patients, on the other hand, delve straight into what's in it for them. Happy patients talk about how you changed their lives. This simply delights their friends and family, who then become potential patients.

The survey extracts these stories so you can bottle them and put them to market. Nothing sells the practice like these stories.

Be sure to survey your team, too. Their perceptions will help you hone in on a rigorous, yet attainable, practice goal. They will help create the story of the practice, too.

The surveys also reveal what media patients use to "shop" for a new dentist. This is important to know so that you invest time and money only on the marketing tactics that will help the practice *now*.

If, for example, you discover that your favorite patients and the people they know aren't following Facebook, then don't invest there. But if every family reads the neighborhood newspaper cover-to-cover, run a print ad there. If 70% of patients pay attention to direct mail, then advertise there.

How to Survey

First, ask each doctor in the practice to list their ten best patients. They are the ones who show up promptly, who articulate their needs, who pay on time, who carry insurance, who follow treatment plans, and who see results. They respect your professional engagement, dental expertise, promptness, and follow-up. These are who you want to replicate in numbers.

Next, craft the questions carefully. Here a few to start:

- What are we doing best?
- What other dental practices did you consider before coming here?
- How are we different from those practices?
- Would you refer friends and family to our practice?
- If so, what would encourage you to do so more often?
- Would you search online for a dental practice like this one?
- If so, what search terms would you use?
- What social media sites do you frequent?
  o Facebook
  o LinkedIn
  o Twitter
  o Other _____
- What types of dental practice marketing do you pay attention to?
  o Website
  o SEO/Online ads
  o Social media
  o Online reviews
  o Direct mail
  o TV/radio
  o Billboards
  o Print ads

Customize the questions and corresponding choices to uncover information that puts marketing in action.

Maybe you are considering foregoing this exercise and jumping directly to launching marketing tactics. Think again.

Lisa of medical device agency Ubiquity uses a similar survey and interview process to formulate targeted marketing for her clients. "Doing homework first will save time and money," she explains. "If you have done your research to find your strategy, you will hit the target rather than shoot in the dark."

Marketing without strategy is like a leaky cauldron. Stemmer says, "You lose two weeks here, two months there from your marketing efforts. Consider how many patient leads, how much production, could have entered the practice in that time with more focus. This brings to light the sheer cost of a lack of focus."

She shares an example. "We got a call from a client who had what I call a bright-shiny-object moment. She had suddenly decided that a brochure was The Thing she needed to jumpstart her revenues. Trouble was, the brochure had absolutely no relationship to the vision and goals of the organization. "I told the client, 'You are doing this for the sheer pleasure of yourself.'"

Marketing just for the sake of marketing seldom works. Always better to market in the name of attracting patients. The most important part: "Once you have created the strategy, you have to embrace it," says Stemmer. "Referring back to it and marketing with consistency will bring the value, not just having it."

If you truly want to grow your practice with a steady flow of the right patients, strategy is the only way to start. "It's like scrubbing in before surgery," says Stemmer. "It's the fundamental start to a complicated procedure."

Surveying first allows you to go to market with a message that is the true essence of your practice, and after time it becomes a self-fulfilling prophecy. Make the same promise across all tactics within your marketing. It's the one promise that you know that you can fulfill every day, the one promise that you become known for – the promise that your patients say you deliver.

Since the promise is derived from the surveys – from the answers to the question, "What are we doing best?" – you can make that promise in the genuine language that patients actually speak. This way it resonates with potential patients who want to know you better. From the moment they enter the door, the entire experience delivers on the promise you made to them. Not only will they come back time and again, but they will also tell others about the practice.

And that cycle means higher production, higher profits, and happier patients – all benefits of the *KABOOM!* method.

CONSTRUCT A MARKETING
MESSAGE AND DESIGN

Once you have asked the right questions of the right people, you will have the data needed to construct a Message and Design Equation that is exclusive to your practice.

The verbatim survey responses lead to the Message and Design Equation. The equation articulates in writing and in pictures what patients love most about the practice.

The equation is: Messaging + Design = Brand.

The brand is the biggest benefit that you are best known for. Volvo is best known as "safe." Coca-Cola is best known as "refreshing." Geico is best known for "savings," as its remarkably memorable gecko constantly reminds us.

What are you best known for?

This is also known as top-of-mind awareness. When you think of tissues, does Kleenex come to mind? When you think of copying does Xerox pop up? There is a reason for that. Those companies have invested millions in helping us recall their name for a particular need at the moment we need it. All others are excluded in our conscious thought.

But you don't need a million-dollar budget to do the same. Here's how to formulate the Message and Design Equation. The key is to depend on the survey results, not your own thoughts and feelings. Consider bringing in an objective third party to assist. Look back through the survey responses for commonalities and trends. Based upon those patterns, complete the worksheet that appears at the end of the book – **Exercise #1: Your Message and Design Equation.**

1. What are three ways that my patients say my practice is different and better than other practices?
2. What is the No. 1 thing people like best about the practice?

As you write out the answer to the first question, the answer to the second one will emerge. The answer to the second question is the Message.

Now ask yourself, "What does this Message look like when translated into Design?"

Here are a few examples...

Example 1

1. What are three ways that my patients say my practice is different and better than other practices?
   - Convenient
   - Approachable
   - Available

2. What is the No. 1 thing people like best about the practice? They feel like this is the go-to downtown dentist.

Message: "Go-to downtown dentist"

Design: Neon colors, photos of city life

Example 2

1. What are three ways that my patients say my practice is different and better than other practices?
   - o Natural
   - o Like me
   - o Trusted experts

2. What is the No. 1 thing people like best about the practice? Most respondents said they have total confidence in themselves and their dentist at this practice.

Message: "Total confidence"

Design: Natural colors, photos of self-assured people

Example 3

1. What are three ways that my patients say my practice is different and better than other practices?
   o Fun to visit
   o Easy appointments
   o Community feeling

2. What is the No. 1 thing people like best about the practice? Patients like that this is dentistry made fun and easy.

Message: "Fun and easy dentistry"
Design: Bright colors with photos of kids in funny dress-up costumes

Once you have articulated Message and Design Equation in the exercise at the end of the book, it remains fixed in place unless the practice changes. If, for example, you acquire another practice or move locations, then run the survey again and redevelop your Message and Design Equation based upon new results.

The Message and Design Equation is an internal tool. It's not something the public will see, but a guide for how the marketing materials should read and look. The Message and Design Equation becomes the starting point for *everything* that is created to market the practice. This way, everything says the same thing and reflects a similar image. Repetition is what makes the unique story memorable.

Now that the Message and Design Equation is locked in, it's time to build the Balanced Marketing Formula for optimum results!

Build a Balanced Marketing Formula

Congratulations! You now have a Marketing and Design Equation, which is more than most dental practices ever do in terms of a marketing method. Now, let's take your strategy a step further.

The Balanced Marketing Formula, or marketing plan, outlines the handful of tactics that are appropriate to take your Message and Design Equation to market. The Balanced Marketing Formula earns higher returns than typical marketing plans because it caters to the target audience's typical media consumption behaviors, and it evenly disperses the marketing budget across all four strategies that drive patient loyalty and patient traffic:

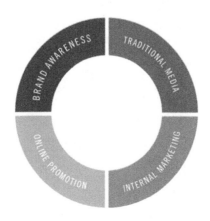

With any Balanced Marketing Formula, there are there are several possible tactics:

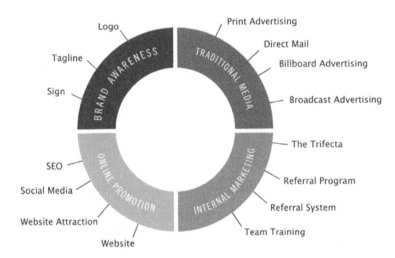

From your survey results, you now know what tactics resonate with your best patients. Just look back over the answers to the question, "What types of dental practice marketing do you pay attention to?" Only a handful of highly targeted tactics will be the focus over the next 12 months. Let the patient surveys show you which ones.

Let's build upon the previous examples.

Example 1
    Message and Design Equation:
    "Go-to downtown dentist" +
    Neon colors, photos of city life
    Balanced Marketing Formula:

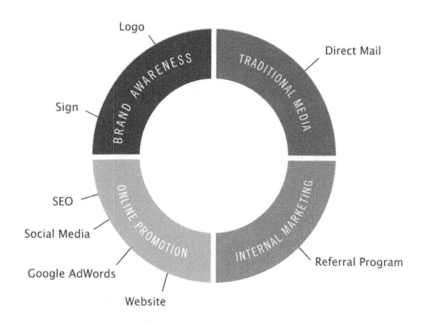

How do we know this is the right Balanced Marketing Formula for this practice? First, since it's new, the practice needed a logo and a sign. Second, the practice is a startup, so direct mail supplemented new patient traffic. Third, it was learned from the surveys that the patients (mostly 20-somethings living downtown) are spending most of their time online, hence the formula is heavy on the online promotion side. Fourth, the practice is not mature enough yet to warrant an internal marketing campaign, which in another year or two may be added to inspire current patients to refer their friends and family.

Example 2
  Message and Design Equation:
  "Total confidence" +
  Natural colors, photos of self-assured people
  Balanced Marketing Formula:

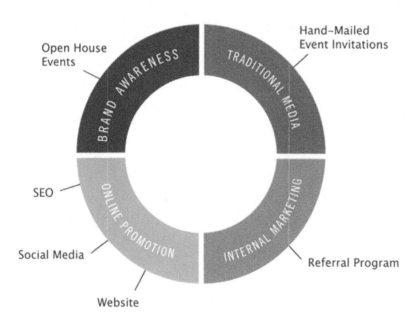

When this practice sent out patient surveys, the dentists learned that their patients were clamoring to refer others. How did they do that? Once every quarter, the practice hosted an open house to thank their most loyal patients and most avid referrers. The invitation envelopes were hand-written to make attendees feel extra special. Then, at every appointment, they handed out incentive cards to call for more referrals. Rather than hitting hard with Google AdWords (which the surveys revealed would be ignored by their patient population), they stuck to more word-of-mouth online marketing through SEO and social media.

Example 3
   Message and Design Equation:
   "Fun and easy dentistry" +
   Bright colors with photos of kids in funny dress-up costumes
   Balanced Marketing Formula:

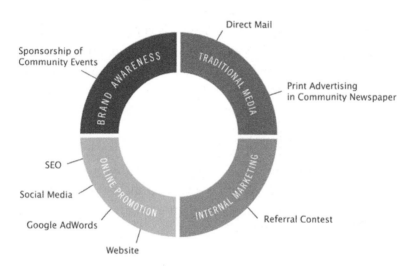

This pediatric dentistry practice is in a community of middle-class and lower-middle class families, and their surveys showed that the community newspaper was a great opportunity for exposure. The dentist had a big goal to double his production rate in a single year, so his Balanced Marketing Formula included eight tactics. Still, the formula remains balanced across all four strategies of marketing.

Each Balanced Marketing Formula will look different because of factors like specialty, community, ideal patient, culture, and vision. Marketing is a living entity that has to shift and grow with the practice.

Yours will also look different. You are unique because no one has your practice's DNA.

The big thing that keeps marketing methodical is the right Balanced Marketing Formula for your unique practice. It may look different next year than it did this year, depending upon ever-shifting goals, trends and budget.

The Balanced Marketing Formula is composed of the strategies and tactics, and inevitably they will overlap. The logo is part of brand awareness, and it will also appear in traditional media and online promotion. A referral program can evolve online just as well as offline. The welcome packet might be downloaded from the website or handed out in person.

Overlap is good. That way, you get the most mileage out of all relevant marketing tactics. Rather than reinventing the wheel each time a marketing initiative is created, always ask, "How can this be used in multiple ways for a higher return on investment?"

Now, let's build your Balanced Marketing Formula.

Tactics

Begin by revisiting the survey responses to all the questions related to marketing tactics, such as these:

- Would you refer friends and family to our practice?
- If so, what would encourage you to do so more often?
- Would you search online for a dental practice like this one?
- If so, what search terms would you use?
- What social media sites to you frequent?
  - o Facebook
  - o LinkedIn
  - o Twitter
  - o Other _____
- What types of dental practice marketing do you pay attention to?
  - o Website
  - o SEO/Online ads
  - o Social media
  - o Online reviews
  - o Direct mail
  - o TV/radio
  - o Billboards
  - o Print ads

Complete the exercise that appears at the end of the book – **Exercise #2: Your Balanced Marketing Formula** – with the names of tactics that are mentioned most often by your survey respondents.

Use the Sample Balanced Marketing Formula at the end of the book for guidance. In that example, the tactics include logo, direct mail, referral mining and website.

•••

Party Responsible

Now, write next to each tactic on your Balanced Marketing Formula the party responsible, or who in the practice will be in charge of executing or managing that tactic.

In the example, the parties responsible include an outside marketer, the office manager, the front desk staff and the dentist.

This is a relatively simple yet critical step. To get any marketing tactic off the ground, it must be assigned to a capable and willing person or group.

•••

Marketing Budget

The next thing to complete on your Balanced Marketing Formula is the marketing budget.

Decide how much to budget for marketing for the year. This is typically 5% to 7% of total annual production. Document your total annual marketing budget in the appropriate area on your Balanced Marketing Formula.

In the example, the practice is on track for $500,000 in annual revenue has budgeted $35,000 a year for marketing, which is 7% of projected gross revenue.

Next, collect estimates from vendors, search out fees online and forecast costs with your team, tactic by tactic. Write down your marketing budget for each tactic on Your Balanced Marketing Formula.

In our example, logo has a budget of $2,500, direct mail has a budget $20,000, referral mining has a budget of $2,500, and website has a budget of $10,000 – all within the total annual marketing budget of $35,000.

If this is your first time deploying a comprehensive marketing strategy, the percentage of initial budget invested may skew higher as the foundation is formed. Startup practices in particular will budget much more than 5% to 7% of projected annual revenue on marketing in the first year – sometimes as much as 50% of projected annual revenue. Once the practice and marketing mature, the budget levels off.

Make no mistake, marketing is fluid. Because it's an ongoing investment, it should constitute a line item on the practice's profit and loss report, just like payroll. And it's an *investment*, not just an expense. And any good investment yields healthy returns.

• • •

Expected ROI

The next step to completing your Balanced Marketing Formula is to forecast the expected ROI, or return on investment.

Consider first each tactic's marketing budget on your Balanced Marketing Formula.

Next, estimate and document the average value of a patient. Average value of a patient for dental practices can be anywhere from $500 to $50,000 per year, depending upon specialty.

In our example, the average value of a patient is $1,500.

Then, estimate how many new patients your Balanced Marketing Formula should attract. Ask each party responsible to provide projected new patients from each tactic. Document the projection on the line labeled expected ROI. Complete the exercise by multiplying the average value of a patient by the projection of acquired patients. Document this dollar figure next to expected ROI by tactic as well. Be sure to fill in the total annual expected ROI, too, including total number of new patients and total dollar figure.

In the example, one of the tactics is direct mail, which has a marketing budget of $20,000 and is expected to yield 120 new patients. Since the average value of a patient is $1,500, that tactic has an expected ROI of $180,000. In all, the example is expected to yield 240 new patients, or $360,000.

Note that in the example, the expected ROI for logo is listed as N/A. As a brand awareness strategy, its success can be difficult to measure. That is why it is one of four tactics in the Balanced Marketing Formula, with the other three being more quantifiable.

Now you are ready to execute the marketing tactics outlined on Your Balanced Marketing Formula. Run all the tactics consistently for six months, and measure results before tweaking anything. As in any experiment, a baseline is needed before the discovery is observed. After the trial period, analyze the reports to see what to continue and what to fix or nix.

• • •

Actual ROI

Your Balanced Marketing Formula is built to be successful, so be sure to measure that success.

Some general ways to measure success may include the practice's reporting on patient and production numbers. In addition to being helpful in gauging the success of the total Balanced

Marketing Formula, these reports can demonstrate the success of brand awareness and internal marketing strategies that are more difficult to measure alone.

For progress reports on online promotions, rely on Google Analytics reporting or other website analytics and social media analytics. There are numerous YouTube videos detailing how get the most out of these reports.

For reporting on traditional media, rely on the vendors. Any reputable direct mail house will be able to provide relevant analytics on a campaign's performance. The same goes for newspaper and magazine representatives as well as television, radio and billboard account executives. Make them prove their success or cut them loose.

To get more granular in measuring actual ROI, consider including custom phone numbers to track calls from particular tactics. This will pinpoint what's working best and what needs fine-tuning to work better.

Advise your front office to always ask and document how new patients found the practice.

In as many ways as possible, try to determine the exact number of patients that came from each tactic. Document this in the actual ROI sections of the Balanced Marketing Formula, including actual ROI for each tactic as well as total actual ROI.

In the example, the direct mail campaign yielded an actual ROI of $168,000, and all tactics together yielded an actual ROI of $345,000.

This will build a record of measurement to return to in six months. If the tactic worked, keep it. If not, alter it and test again. If it's still not working in another six months, ditch it. But give it time, and be patient. While it may not catch on in month six, it may take off in month eight.

• • •

Now you have surveyed patients and team members, constructed a Message and Design Equation, and built a Balanced Marketing Formula. This is the foundation for the *KABOOM!* method. These tools will allow you to experiment and get creative with marketing while still adhering to guidelines for success. This is the best way to launch the most effective marketing tactics.

You are ready to deploy your Balanced Marketing Formula, tactic by tactic. Get ready for enduring results!

Top 10 Common Mistakes in Setting the Foundation

1. **Experimenting without a hypothesis.** Instead, set a goal first. Expect the *KABOOM!* method to produce measurable results such as an uptick in patients seen per month or in annual production. With a goal in mind, you can clearly measure success.
2. **Doing what's popular.** Rather than throwing money at online marketing because it's trendy, invest only in the marketing tactics that make most sense for your practice.
3. **Too many scientists in the lab.** Stick to two or three key decision-makers who will be with you throughout the whole process. Avoid crowdsourcing, which is gathering anecdotal opinions, as this is more harmful that helpful in a strategic environment.
4. **Going it alone.** By contrast, a lack of collaboration can be equally detrimental. Let the happiest patients tell the practice story rather than trying to write it in a vacuum. This process will prevent you from getting too technical in your marketing communications. Plus, a small team of

two or three colleagues will help you think creatively and stay on track.

5. **Re-experimenting too soon.** Once you discover the Balanced Marketing Formula, test those tactics for a good six months before changing or adding tactics. It takes that long to tell if the experiment is working. Patience, patience, patience!

6. **Letting your own opinion rule.** What your patients think about the practice trumps what you think. Rely on their input to *objectively* build the Message and Design Equation.

7. **Feature focusing.** Turn your attention to benefits instead. Highlight what your patients love most about *you*, not technology or too much clinical detail.

8. **Spending not investing.** Be careful not to spend too much on marketing. If, after six months, any tactic is not producing a return on investment, nix it. Returns are not always in the form of dollars. Added exposure and awareness in front of the people who matter most can be a very healthy investment. Again, adhere to the budget.

9. **Lack of documentation.** The foundation will erode – and fast – unless it's articulated in writing. Finish the exercises provided at the end of the book to be sure you have all the documentation you need for marketing success.

10. **Perfectionism.** Now that you have a method behind marketing, there may be the tendency to overthink things. Set deadlines. Consider the idea that 90% done is done. Have a team member keep you accountable for finishing projects within a certain timeframe. And by the way, have fun!

PART TWO

BRAND AWARENESS

Now that you have surveyed patients and team members, constructed a Message and Design Equation, and built a Balanced Marketing Formula, it's time to deploy the marketing, tactic by tactic.

Part Two demonstrates how to deploy brand awareness tactics like logo, tagline and sign – if they appear in your Balanced Marketing Formula.

Brand awareness is all about staying "top of mind." When it comes to brand awareness efforts, it can be difficult to test each of these tactics, analyze data, draw conclusions, and track results. This is why it is critical that brand awareness tactics be part of the Balanced Marketing Formula, which will include more measurable tactics.

Let's dive in!

THE SCIENCE BEHIND THE LOGO

Perhaps you don't yet have a logo. Or you need a new logo after an acquisition or transition. Or maybe the survey responses revealed that it's time to redesign the logo. If logo is a tactic in your Balanced Marketing Formula, here are simple instructions on how to design the logo that's right for you.

Let's start with the anatomy of several types of logos:

1. **Custom Font Only** – FedEx is a well-known example. This font (or typeface) is memorable for its bold, blocky letters, and it includes a hidden arrow to convey motion. The custom font is not the standard Arial or Times New Roman, but a unique typeface that stands for dependable shipping. There is nothing else to the logo other than the letters of the brand name. In the wellness world, Zantac, CVS Pharmacy, and Johnson & Johnson are Custom Font Only logos. They work best for organizations with highly memorable names.

2. **Mark Plus Font** – Starbucks is the most ubiquitous example. We all know the white siren, or twin-tailed mermaid, that harkens back to the coffeemaker's origins in

seafaring Seattle. She appears inside of a green circle – that's the "mark." Around the mark originally appeared the words "Starbucks Coffee" – that's the font. (The company has dropped the words since the mark is now recognizable on its own, like the Target bull's eye.) In healthcare, Blue Cross, Mayo Clinic, and American Red Cross have Mark Plus Font logos. It's a great way for an organization to communicate through word and image who they are.

3. **Initial Plus Font** – Everyone knows the McDonald's golden arches, that ubiquitous "M." The mark is the first initial of the brand name. Initial Plus Font logos in health and wellness include the universal blue "H" that provides roadside directions to hospitals, ADA for the American Dental Association, and AARP for the American Association of Retired Persons. The Initial Plus Font logo is best for the organization that has a lot of brand equity built into its name; in other words, the name has been in use for many years and is easily recognized by the entire community. Think *NY* for New York Yankees.

When it comes to choosing a font, there are a number of options. Notice that this book is written in a Serif Font, in which each letter has small lines or tiny feet on its end.

Serif Fonts with feet are typically used in long-form writing because they are regarded as more legible for the time it takes to read a piece. Newspapers and magazines use Serif Fonts in their body copy. In a logo, a Serif Font can convey longevity and stability. It can also make a longer brand name easier to read. Favorite Serif Fonts for logos include:

Garamond

Baskerville

Georgia

By contrast, the fonts below use a Sans Serif Font. "Sans" is French for "without." The Sans Serif Font is without feet. Sans Serif Fonts most often appear in headlines and short-format writing because they grab the reader's attention. A Sans Serif Font conveys modernity and lightness for a dental practice. It makes a short brand name pop out. Top picks for Sans Serif Fonts include:

Helvetica

Optima

Futura

Think of the logo process as trying on hats. Once you find the right structure for your hat, you can begin to customize the shapes, colors, accents, and other details. The goal for the design is to appeal to patients and potential patients rather than your own personal preference.

Now let's get into the design process. First, look back at the Message and Design Equation. Think about what you want to communicate visually that will convey what you have written. What shapes come to mind? What two or three colors? What objects come to mind? Consider common objects such as plants, animals, foods, letters and numbers that are universally recognizable and therefore memorable.

Get creative, even so far as to become abstract. Once you think of a few objects that best represent the Message and Design Equation, ask yourself, "What is a new and different way to show this in a way that fits with my equation?"

Sketch out on paper ideas that come to mind. There is no bad idea at this point. Just put ideas you can think of down on paper. Afterward, sort out and select the strongest options. Circle the favorites. Cross off any that rank lower on the Message and Design Equation. Stick to the process. The logo options will be spot-on if they reflect your Message and Design Equation. They feel right in your gut.

Present the strongest sketch ideas to two or three of your team members. Keep the pool small. Start by sharing with them the Message and Design Equation, and explain that the logo must represent this equation. Stress that this is less a matter of opinion and more a strategic process. Show them the proposed logos. With the team's help, narrow it down to the two strongest ideas.

Now you have two logo semifinalists. You can turn the sketches over to a graphic designer to create both logos for final consideration.

Or you can design them yourself. Start by scanning the sketches into a computer. At this stage, it is good to more fully explore different variations on font and color. Give both logos a color palette, preferably each a different one. Be sure the colors match the Message and Design Equation. Keep refining until you and the team feel like the logos are finished.

Don't get discouraged. Fortune 500 companies spent millions formulating their logos through research, focus groups and surveys. You are doing the very same thing, but at considerably less cost.

When you see the logo for the first time it will be all alone on the page. The patient typically sees logos in the context of something bigger, as part of a website or a sign. Once you lock in the logo and colors, it will really come to life in your business card, mailer or other marketing tactics.

The last thing to do is print the two finished logos in large format, tape them to your front door, stand back, and see which one feels best.

Choose your logo!

KABOOM! Logo development is no longer a mystery. It's a method.

ADDING A TAGLINE

Once your logo is complete, consider whether a tagline is needed. The tagline is necessary when the practice name alone does not articulate what it does or its value offered. Think of it as a motto or a slogan to clarify the mission succinctly.

For example, the practice name *Town Center Dentistry & Orthodontics* says what they *do*, but there is no value proposition. Their surveys revealed that they are best known for their genuine approach to care, so they added the tagline "Genuine Care. Life-Changing Results." This clarifies their value to patients.

The practice name of *Dr. Thomas S. Jennings* is so basic that it may require a tagline to demonstrate what it does *and* its value. His surveys showed that patients know him best for his commitment to comfort and excellence, so he added the tagline "Committed to Comfort and Excellence in Dentistry." This offers clarity on both issues.

The tagline is based upon the Message and Design Formula, and answers the question: What does it do at what value? It provides excellent name recognition when it works. Think: Nothing runs like a Deere, Johnny on the Spot, Diamonds are Forever. A plumbing service in Kentucky boasts a clever poker analogy, "A Flush Beats A Full House."

A tagline isn't based on conjecture. It's based on the *KABOOM!* method.

A Technique for Signs

If signage is one of the tactics on the Balanced Marketing Formula, here is a technique for the sign design.

Begin by researching whether the landlord or property owner's association has any restrictions. Keep in mind that any obstructions of view that will need to be overcome.

With those parameters in mind, consider where exterior signage is needed – perhaps on the exterior door, on the area above the entrance, or on the outside wall of the building. Signage may need to appear in multiple areas. Consider as well where interior signage will be required – maybe way-finding signs in the building lobby, on an interior door, or behind the front desk.

Negotiate price discounts with the signage installer when you order multiple signs at once.

Next, sketch on paper all that comes to mind pertaining to the signage. The logo will be the foundation. What else is needed? A tagline? Directional arrow? Lighting? Outdoor signage will need adequate lighting to be visible at night and will also need to be made of materials that will withstand the elements.

Refine the sketches. Select the stronger option to send to the sign company. Require that they send a proof of the sign before installation. Ask the vendor to Photoshop the mockup onto an image of the actual area where it will be installed. Ask for front and side views of the mockups to get a complete perspective.

Once you approve the mockups, the installer should provide final schematics and secure any required permits for installation. The only thing left is make sure signage is delivered and quality-checked.

Ta da! You have signs!

No more guesswork – just the *KABOOM!* method.

Top 10 Common Mistakes in Brand Awareness

1. **Being unimaginative.** Skip the standard font for the logo, like Arial or Times New Roman, in favor of getting creative with a custom or lesser-known font that best represents you.
2. **Jumping the gun.** Share logo or sign designs only after you have finalized them with the core team, but not while they are still under development.
3. **Stroking the ego.** As you proceed through logo and sign development, suspend the urge to design in your favorite color. Use instead colors and images that resonate with so many favorite patients.
4. **Defaulting to the obvious.** In logo or sign development, avoid using obvious objects like teeth or dental instruments. Experiment instead with objects that every person can relate to, your patients most importantly. Be creative!
5. **Cutting costs at all costs.** Online graphic design marketplaces are all the rage. They will design your logo for

as little as $5. To have them design the logo or anything else without the *KABOOM!* method would be unscientific, and therefore unreliable. Plus, you get what you pay for. Stick to your Marketing Budget.

6. **Sensational branding.** Resist the urge toward "sensational," or intentionally misspelled, branding. Think Blu-ray, Cheez-It, and Dunkin' Donuts. Also known as "divergent" spelling, sensational spelling is hardly advised for professionals for fear of trivializing the practice. Can you imagine While-U-Wait Pediatric Dentistry?

7. **Overdoing a good thing.** Many logos lose their power because their typeface is hard to read or muddled. There's a fine line between being clever and too cute. Aim for a logo that is memorable, simple, and easy to read.

8. **Incomplete statement.** Together, an effective logo and a good tagline complete a sentence. They say what the practice is at what value to whom. If the logo doesn't make the whole statement, add a tagline.

9. **Expecting measureable results.** Results from brand awareness tactics are nearly impossible to measure. Instead, measure results against the whole Balanced Marketing Formula.

10. **Not investing.** Brand awareness tactics go a long way in terms of demonstrating the practice's value to potential patients. Be sure to allot a portion of Marketing Budget to brand awareness for steady overall results from the Balanced Marketing Formula.

PART THREE

TRADITIONAL MEDIA

Traditional media has gotten a bum rap ever since the so-called Age of Empowerment in advertising and marketing. Many dentists are under the false impression that everything today is happening online, and they neglect to balance their marketing formula by including this critical strategy.

Almost all practices benefit from deploying a few tactics in traditional media. If brand awareness is about staying top of mind, traditional media is about remaining front and center.

Consider your survey results to see which traditional media tactics are right for your practice. Did patients remember seeing that last direct mail piece? Do they see billboards around town? Do they read the community newspaper or city magazine? Do they have a favorite radio or television station?

Remember the allotment of Marketing Budget that you assigned to traditional media? There is a common misperception that traditional media can be expensive or have low returns compared to Online Marketing. In fact, a direct mail campaign can lead to an immediate spike in patient traffic precisely when needed, and that sends revenue to the bottom line. The objective is to return to the foundation you set for the *KABOOM!* method to create the traditional media mix that will work best.

Media buys are often negotiated and always discounted for volume. When you are ready to purchase, ask the account rep for the rate sheet, which will show the cost of the media reduced over the number of times it runs. The longer the run, the lower the rate.

Sometimes one rep can purchase media for you across a variety of media such as billboards and radio all in one.

Be sure to ask if they offer online marketing to complement your traditional media tactics. Some newspaper reps, for example, will run your ad in the print *and* web editions at no additional cost.

Part Three will explore how to get the most out of traditional media with the four tactics of direct mail, print advertising, billboard advertising, and broadcast advertising.

Direct Mail Debunked

The first indication that your practice can benefit from direct mail is that the surveys validate that it has worked in the past.

Direct mail works great if competition is fierce and you need to secure a foothold in the market. It positions you as a resource of genuine value to your community by programming the immediate surrounding population to think of you first above others, *and* to perceive you a certain way.

Direct mail can be a hefty investment, and it can really pay off. That said, this tactic is best outsourced to an expert.

According to Shayne Harris of EOS Corporate, a dental direct marketing agency, 80% of patients come to a typical practice from a radius of one to three miles. Direct mail targets that circle.

Harris likens direct mail to an adrenaline rush. It supports the health and lifespan of the practice by injecting a steady shot of advertising each time a mailer "drops," or is mailed out. This tactic is great for practices that need an immediate boost in patient traffic or to capture quick returns.

"There is three-week window of effectiveness for each drop," Harris explains. "95% of the return comes in this timeframe."

If a doctor is planning to sell a practice, Harris recommends using direct mail to boost the patient count over the three years prior to transitioning, then selling based upon the projected earnings.

To be sure, each adrenaline rush is followed by a dip. That is why it's important to embrace repetition and to supplement direct mail with the other tactics in the Balanced Marketing Formula. "Repetition builds reputation," Harris reminds us.

"Direct mail is formulaic," he adds. "There is no happenstance." When developing a direct mail campaign, he recommends that you first qualify and quantify your market. Paint the picture of your ideal patient mix and what they might have in common: affluent retirees, avid skiers, stay-at-home parents, $100,000 income, recently bought a boat. The list goes on. The more granular the picture, the better focused the campaign.

"A reputable direct mail house will correlate that information with their analytics to target a very specific type of person to attract to the practice," says Harris.

Have a look at your Marketing Budget, and share with your direct mail vendor the amount you have allotted to this tactic. Confine the vendor to an effective campaign within that budget. Be sure to adhere to your goal, quantifying how many new patients you need from the campaign to achieve the desired return on investment.

Before pulling the trigger, ask how the vendor will identify results. A custom phone number can track which new patient calls originated from which mailer. The vendor should report after each drop a demographic breakdown of how many households were hit.

Particularly in this marketing tactic, it is imperative that you stick to your Message and Design formula. The value and offer have to be crystal clear, or the effort is fruitless. As Harris puts it, "In direct mail, when you don't know what to say, you tend to say everything and you end up saying nothing." Don't try to cram ten pounds of text into a five-pound mailer.

A direct mail vendor can help guide you through the creative process to develop the most effective campaign for your practice. Direct mail experts have a specific formula for crafting the right pieces within any given campaign. Moreover, they design each piece to keep the eye moving to all the critical areas in just a few seconds. All of this drives results by making a compelling offer.

The secret mix creates a high level of interest. The mailer should motivate the reader to take the next step, not divulge all the information at once.

A direct mail piece is dead in the water without an offer. Without an incentive, you leave your prospect hanging. The offer is nothing more than a motivator to get the patient to take action.

Here are a couple of examples of compelling direct mailers that worked well in attracting the right patients to the respective practices:

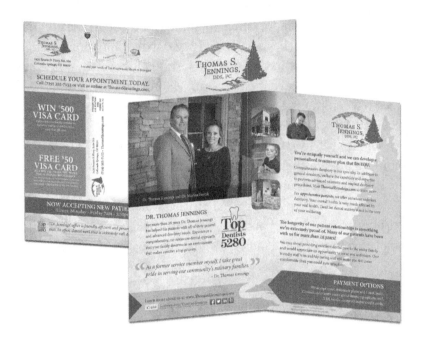

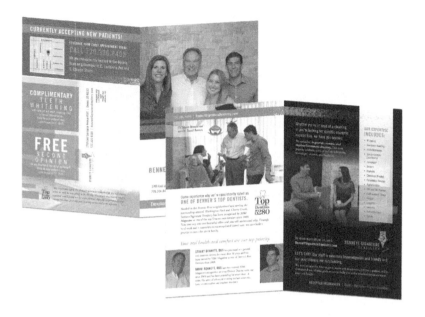

In formulating your offer, bear in mind that discounting fees in direct mail tends to turn the practice into a commodity and can diminish the perceived value of the practice. The offer doesn't have to include a discount, but it does need to be valuable to the potential patient. Offering a free initial consultation, for example, is not discounting your services, it's opening a door.

Be sure the phone number is large and legible on the direct mailer. That's the next step you want them to take – call for an appointment.

Use this as a guide for working with the right direct mail vendor, and you will get more patients from this tactic.

When backed by the *KABOOM!* method, direct mail can work wonders!

PRINT ADVERTISING STRATEGY

Print advertising may likely appear in your Balanced Marketing Formula. Perhaps this is because your surveys show that your patients are avid readers of the community newspaper or a particular magazine. Or because you have tested print advertising in the past and determined that it delivers a strong return on investment.

Or maybe it's because the surveys indicated that your patients are not big users of online media. One dental practice was like a sorority for wealthy women. The ladies would hang out there, even if they didn't need medical attention. "I think they like the escape," the doctor told me. These women regularly referred new patients to the dentist, and they all read the neighborhood newspaper cover-to-cover. Online marketing didn't make any sense for her practice. A long-run print ad did instead.

Here's what you need to know about print advertising to make it work for you. Let's look first at the anatomy of a print ad that drives results.

The best print ads tell a story. The object is not to inform ad nauseam, but to inspire. Keep reminding yourself that no one can tell your practice's story like your happiest patients. With written patient consent for HIPAA compliance, consider creating a print ad campaign that features testimonials from patients, like the example shown here:

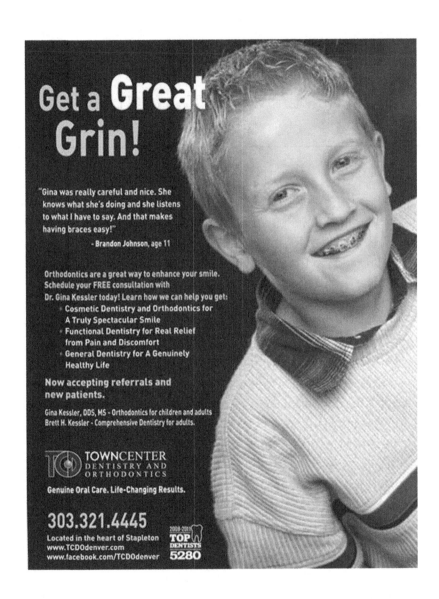

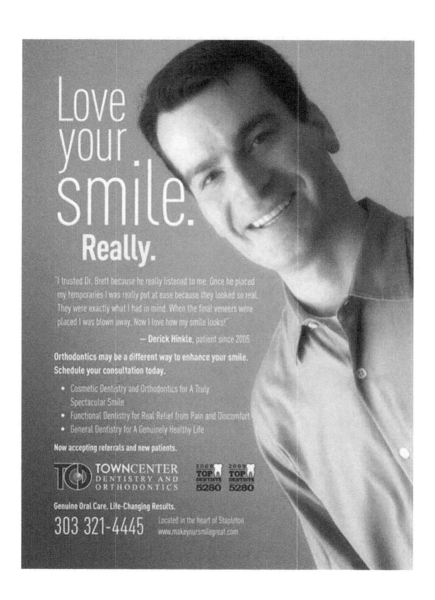

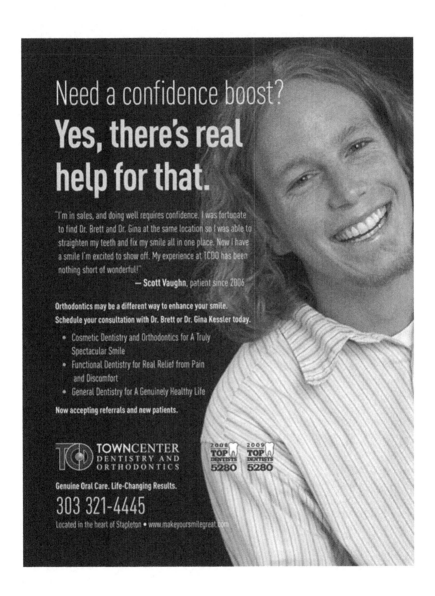

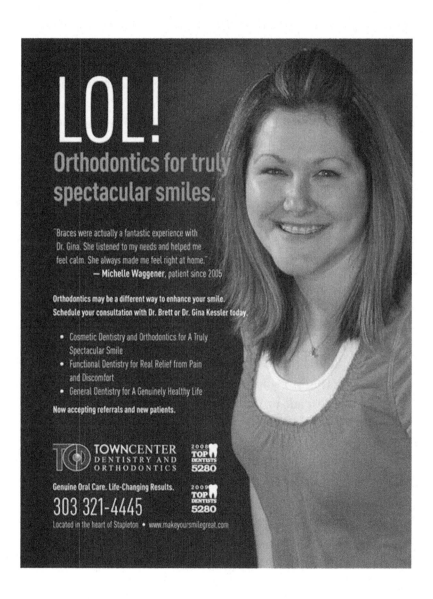

A strong print ad has a short, eye-catching headline. As mentioned in The Science Behind the Logo in Part Two, a Sans Serif Font is more legible. Avoid using the practice name or logo for the headline. That would be like walking into a crowded room and announcing, "I'm Dr. John Smith!" Instead, use a clever phrase to draw the reader in. Once you pique their interest, they will find your name and contact details, which should appear toward the bottom of the ad design.

People are visual creatures. Lighten up on the text and go big with an appealing and relevant graphic. Avoid staid stock photography in favor of custom professional shots of your team, a patient or your office space. Go with what's inviting to the potential patient, not necessarily your favorite shots.

Be sure to use high-resolution photography and convert each image to a TIFF file that is bigger than 40MB, or a JPEG larger than 6MB. The term "resolution" refers to the detail in an image. The greater the detail, the more crisply it will reproduce in print. Low-resolution photos are fine for use on the web, but print always requires high-resolution imagery.

The very best ads provide an "aha!" moment or get a chuckle. Get creative and include a clever and memorable twist to your ad. Ask the publication to run it upside down occasionally, and include a small disclaimer at the bottom – or in this case, top – saying "Intentionally run upside down." Use a popular phrase to rope people in. "Leaks Like a Sieve" was the headline for a roofing company ad that ran for a long time, and while I haven't seen the ad in years I still remember it because it made me laugh.

Be sure to include a compelling call-to-action. This is the equivalent to the direct mail offer. Incentivize the reader to take the next step. *Free whitening for life. New-patient gift.*

Complimentary consultation. Then tell the reader exactly how to take the next step. *Call today. Make an appointment. Email for more information.* Be sure that clear contact information appears in the ad. At the very least, that means phone number and web address.

As with all traditional media, consistency is key. Run the same campaign at least 10 times in the same publication to be noticed, and even longer to be *remembered.* In the case just cited, the above four ads constitute one campaign, or series of similarly designed ads, all working toward the same goal.

With a dynamic print ad strategy backed by the *KABOOM!* method, new patient traffic will level out rather than swing up and down each month.

BLUEPRINT FOR BILLBOARD ADVERTISING

Billboard advertising is likely in your Balanced Marketing Formula if your surveys validated this tactic, and if you aim to reach a vast and diverse population across a particular neighborhood or metropolitan area.

You may want to advertise on multiple billboards around town to achieve the greatest reach. This marketing tactic can require a significant investment of $1,000 a month or as much as $1,000 a week for each billboard. Be sure it's what's best for reaching your goals. Under the right circumstances, it can be a good way to regularly attract a large number of patients to the practice.

Billboards work best when they run in conjunction with other traditional media efforts. The message on the billboard matches the one running in the city magazine ads, which matches the jingle playing every Tuesday morning on the radio during rush hour. It all ties together.

Billboards are not just signs along the highway. Many city centers feature brightly illuminated digital billboards that were first made popular in Times Square. Large-format advertising on the side of city buses and metro rail systems may gain more attention than their stationary counterparts.

Pith is the essence of billboard messaging. You have only a split second to grab the eye and share one concept. Sukle, an advertising agency in Denver, nailed pith and brevity with their billboards for Denver Water. The campaign was so clever that the trade journal AdWeek featured it as exemplary. Read more about it at www.adweek.com/topic/denver-water.

The anatomy of a billboard that drives results is simple: Headline, no more than eight words, followed by logo. That's it. You don't even have to include your phone number or website. If your billboard is catchy enough, they will search you out from just your practice name.

Billboards for medical promotions are tough to write. Here's one for a hospital under construction: "Keep your eyes on the road, we are not open yet."

Short format is the most difficult to write. As Mark Twain famously put it, "I didn't have time to write a short letter." To write a catchy billboard, make it a game with your team to come up with as many clever, funny phrases of 5-8 words that tie back to your Message and Design Equation.

Eventually the winners will emerge and your billboard campaign will be launched. And any billboard campaign grounded in the *KABOOM!* method will yield more regular results.

FOOLPROOF BROADCAST ADVERTISING

Perhaps it was revealed on your surveys that broadcast advertising, or television and radio ads, should appear in your Balanced Marketing Formula.

Broadcast ads work very well with billboards to provide wide-reaching awareness across a particular community. Like billboard advertising, television and radio ads require a significant investment, so be sure to budget wisely. When done right, these ads pack the power to attract masses of new patients, so the returns can be quite healthy.

Writing and producing television and radio ads is complicated, so it's best left to the experts. With this type of traditional media, a rep who can write the ad copy can also have the spot recorded with professional voiceover and actors.

A television or radio commercial is often referred to as a "spot." Hold your rep accountable for creating a top-notch spot for you with the following guidelines.

1. Begin by sharing your Brand and Messaging Formula with your rep.

2. Ask to see the suggested script before the spot is produced, and be sure that the writing reflects your Brand

and Messaging Formula. Humor works very well in broadcast advertising, but only if it fits your practice. Emotional appeals can also work well, but shy away from fear-based advertising.

3. As with other traditional media, the offer is the key element. Make sure the offer and the contact information are clearly articulated. In broadcast advertising, it can work to your advantage to have the contact information repeated several times in the spot for easy recall. Listeners or viewers often have mobile devices in hand while consuming your message, so there's no better time to get them to act than *right now*.

4. A vanity phone number or memorable website address goes a long way in broadcast advertising. 1-800-DENTIST is a great example of how this works in advertising. The number is so memorable that on radio they say it only once, and in television ads they show it only once.

5. A jingle, or short tune including the practice name and phone number, can also help with recall. A jingle works best when the name is short and easy to sing. If using a jingle, be sure to use the same jingle for *every* ad produced. Consistency is key when tapping recall.

6. Use the same voiceover or acting talent for added memorability. Allison Janney is the voice behind every one of Kaiser Permanente's broadcast ads, both television and radio. TMZ describes her voice as "so soothing that it can make even the worst of news seem okay."

7. After the ad is scripted, the rep will get it recorded or produced. Review the final ad with the three Ds in mind: distinctive, digestible, and deed-oriented. It is distinctive when it reflects your Brand and Messaging Formula and

sets you apart from the competition. It is digestible when it tells one cohesive story that is easy to understand and clearly articulated. It's also deed-oriented when it asks the listener or viewer act, to take the next step, and extends a carrot to induce them to do so.

8. As with print and billboard advertising, extended campaigns work better than a single ad. Once you and your rep develop the first great ad, have the rep develop it into at least a three-part series. A campaign tells a bigger story and paints a clearer picture.

You can have faith in your broadcast advertising approach knowing that it's anchored in the *KABOOM!* method.

Top 10 Common Mistakes in Traditional Media

1. **Ignoring Traditional Media.** Resist the notion that traditional media is passé. Most dental practices can benefit from investing some portion of their marketing budget into these tactics to stay front and center.
2. **One and Done.** Avoid the urge to run one advertisement or mail a single postcard. Generally speaking, a prospect has to read/see/hear an offer ten times for it even to be noticed, let alone acted upon. Repetition is key to all traditional media. Even better, repetition across traditional media tactics can propel the practice to ubiquity. Besides, campaigns are always better than single efforts. How many times did you see the promo for a TV show before you tuned in?
3. **"Don't confuse informative with persuasive,"** says Shayne Harris. This goes not just for direct mail, but also for print and billboard advertising as well as broadcast advertising. Less is more. Go for pith and punch.

4. **Dismemberment.** Don't show teeth-only shots as part of the traditional media tactics. They are eerie to the non-dental population. Show only full-face shots to illustrate transformation. Even then, tread lightly. "Before" photos that may be considered frightening to laypeople should be eliminated.

5. **Trifold brochures.** The standard trifold brochure is dated. Instead, invest in a welcome packet. It's like the sexy booklet that car dealers give out when you visit for a test drive. The welcome packet is engaging, sharable and gives new patients the feeling, "Wow, I belong here!"

6. **Sponsorships.** It seems that everywhere you turn, community organizations are asking dental practices to sponsor something. *Advertise at the community ballpark. Give out free toothbrushes to the entire fifth grade. By a booth at the local 5K run.* The worst example is to participate in the neighborhood co-op door-to-door flyer that includes the logo of every business in the area. You will get lost in the clutter. It's always good to give back, so pick one sponsorship opportunity for the year. Beyond that, most of your advertising is better spent on direct marketing and high-visibility awareness rather than these limited-impact initiatives.

7. **Phone directories.** Dex and Yellow Pages have amazing salespeople and some intriguing online products to supplement the listing in their outdated books, but your money is better spent elsewhere. Get a simple, free listing – that's it. If you are currently running a phone directory ad, measure the cost per year with the number of new patients you can trace to that ad. If it's not providing

a healthy return, cancel it and put your resources where they will really count.

8. **Low-balling on business card and stationery.** With your logo in hand from the brand awareness phase, be sure to get a well-designed business card, letterhead and envelope for the practice. Many everyday traditional media tactics will require it, like patient agreement forms, faxes and the occasional press release.

9. **Stopping short.** Radio and television ads should be repurposed on your website and in your social media. This stuff is online gold. Web users love little sound bites and short videos. Plus, the better your ads, the more apt they are to be shared or even to go viral across the web.

10. **Failure to proof.** Once your traditional media hits the streets, there's no turning back. An ad in Houston hit 500,000 households reading ABORTION ATTORNEY. They meant *adoption* attorney. If a mistake or typo leaks out there, it's nowhere near as easy or inexpensive to correct as with online efforts. Be sure to proofread the ad copy carefully.

PART FOUR

ONLINE PROMOTION

Online promotion is all the rage these days. Facebook, Twitter, Instagram, Google, Bing, Yahoo! – they're fun to say, they're hot, and a lot of doctors are clamoring to be all over them.

Why?

We are a gadget-obsessed culture, and there's no greater gadget than the World Wide Web. The web is the only form of media that give us so much individual *control*. People can become a blogger or a published author overnight. Order that new book online right now and start reading it on your tablet immediately. Amazon.com is talking about a drone that will deliver wares in 30 minutes or less, like a pizza. Hired a new employee? No problem. Just log in to your website and upload her photo and bio. Instant gratification never felt so right.

"Marketing" companies have sprouted up everywhere, offering to "get you found at the top of Google" or "manage your online reputation," or "remove negative reviews."

Plus, there is a lingering belief that online promotion is far less expensive than traditional media. In the early days, online promotion was commonly thought of as free. Just jump online, post your information and get instant exposure in front of potential patients.

If only it were that easy.

A Balanced Marketing Formula includes online promotion *among other strategies.* It can be easy to get carried away with the online craze by overinvesting. So much online promotion is designed to be do-it-yourself that it's easy to bite off too much. The Balanced Marketing Formula keeps you on track and on budget.

Be sure that the marketing budget allots an appropriate percentage to online promotions. Not too high, not too low – refer back to your Balanced Marketing Formula at the end of Part One to be sure of the right investment for your practice. While many online promotions can be done on your own, you will need a vendor's help with certain tactics to really see results. For example, it is possible to launch a Google AdWords campaign on one's own, but that would be like your patient performing her own root canal. Some procedures are better left to the experts.

Go back to the survey results to understand which online promotions to focus on. What do people like about your website, and what can you improve? Are your patients and their peers searching online for their healthcare needs? Are your potential patients frequent Facebook posters, or do they prefer LinkedIn?

In Part Four, you will see how to get the most out of your online promotions, including website, social media, search exposure, and reputation management.

Disciplined Website Design

Let's say the surveys indicated that your website needs a makeover. Keep it simple. A 15-page website is really all you need for a one- to two-dentist private practice. One of those pages can be the blog, which will fill in with entries over time and enhance the content of the website. Like your marketing on the whole, your website is a living organism. Rich, relevant content and frequent updates are what make a website visible on search engines – not content overdose. Quality trumps quantity.

If you bristled at the word "blog" in the previous paragraph, fear not. A blog is nothing more than an online journal. Excerpts of published medical articles, conversations with other physicians, and muses on your work all make interesting and easy-to-formulate fodder. Don't carry the weight alone. Some of entries can come from your own writings, and then pick up other sources to round it out. Search online for expert material that can be reposted, but be sure it's properly credited. Have staff write guest blog entries about what it's like to work at the practice. Invite a patient to write up what it's like to be under your care. This takes the pressure off and makes your blog credible rather than egotistical. Post once a week and your blog will grow over time.

Be sure that the website provides an "action opportunity" on every page. *Call for an appointment. Fill out this form to learn more. Follow the practice on Facebook. Enter an email address and get a free care guide.* Each person who arrives to the website will have different preferences, so provide a number of options. The more options, the more likely web visitors are to act and thereby stay engaged with the practice.

The website should be designed to whet the appetite and encourage action. Be sure that the web text and look matches the Message and Design Equation and is promotional rather than informational.

My friend Dr. Cote shared with me the three A's of websites that drive results: affability, ability and availability. It's tough to say where he picked these up, as the concept is all over the web and could very well be applied to developing a successful medical practice on the whole.

A powerful website makes the practice look *affable,* or likeable. Visitors should see warm and inviting photos of the office, doctors and staff. They should get the feeling, "I might like them. They could earn my trust."

A great website makes it clear that the physicians are highly *able.* It should be clear in the first few seconds of looking at the home page any of the dentists' awards and accolades and any compelling before-and-after cases they have completed. Visitors should get the feeling, "They seem capable. They would take good care of me."

A terrific website articulates that the dentist is *available.* Office hours, address and directions should appear on every page. This conveys the feeling, "It would be easy for me to at least check them out. I could make it happen."

Some sources add a fourth: affordability. In marketing, selling on price is rarely a good idea, which is why it's not included here. *50% off today, lower teeth whitening only!* Eek!

Website development can be a lot like building a home: It's a big undertaking and a huge investment; it opens up high probability of scope, time and budget creep; and the finished product is a public reflection of you, which means it has to be *just so*.

Use these eight milestones to help guide your provider to completion:

1. Budget. Share with your web developer the budget you have allotted to this tactic, and execute a written agreement stipulating those terms.

2. Sitemap. This is the blueprint for the website. The web developer should outline in text the navigation of the site, demonstrate the page flow, and show the titles of all pages that will be developed. Be sure that you both fully agree on the sitemap before proceeding. After you approve a blueprint, the construction begins. Adding a room on a house (or adding a webpage) can drive up costs.

3. Web Text. Next, request that your provider write, edit and proof all copy or text to appear on the website. Share your Message and Design Equation to eliminate the guesswork and streamline the process. Be sure to lock in the web text before going to the next step. Just as a bathroom with one sink has a different configuration than a bathroom with two, so too do your webpages shift with more or less text.

4. Wireframe. Ask for a basic layout in black-and-white of the functionality of the website. Will there be a large

"slider" of compelling images on the home page? Where will images appear and where will text appear? Where will action opportunities appear? Be sure to see a "wireframe" for the home page and at least one other page. This part of the process is like the newly framed home. You begin to see what it will be like when it's finished. Refine and sign off on the wireframe to go to the most exciting part: the actual build-out.

5. Homepage Design. Focus on the homepage first. This way, you can see the heart of the home nearly finished before all of the other rooms are designed. As with everything else, be sure that the homepage design correlates with your Message and Design Equation. Approving this will set the rest of the build out in motion.

6. Website Development. The rest of the webpages should be developed from the foundation set in steps 2 through 5. This may be a good step to outsource to an expert. The foundation locks in the direction for the rest of the design, making the development process much faster and more exciting. Rather than build a separate mobile site, which was a popular solution in the early 2010s, have your provider build the website to be *responsive*. This means the website will automatically resize to various screen sizes (phone, tablet, laptop, desktop). The content will be digestible regardless of where it appears.

7. Testing. Prior to launch, be sure that functionality is tested across all browsers and devices to ensure quality display regardless of who's viewing it.

8. Launch!

It's key to remember that your website is nothing more than a billboard in the middle of the ocean until you make the effort to attract visitors with tactics like social media, search engine optimization (SEO), Google AdWords and more. These are the tactics that transform your practice website into an efficient machine that attracts visitors to your site and patients into your door while you focus on what you do best. That's the *KABOOM!* method for you!

DEMYSTIFYING SOCIAL MEDIA

In 2009 the Social Media Revolution video hit YouTube and went viral, scaring the socks off the millions of people who saw it. (Source: https://www.youtube.com/watch?v=sIFYPQjYhv8)

"Is social media a fad?" the video challenges. "Or is it the biggest shift since the Industrial Revolution?" The video explodes with startling statistics set to heart-thumping music:

- If Facebook were a country, it would be the world's 3rd largest.
- 80% of companies are using LinkedIn as their primary tool to find employees.
- Generation X and Y consider email passé, and some universities have stopped distributing email addresses. Instead, they are distributing eReaders, iPads, and tablets.
- 78% of consumers trust peer recommendations, while only 14% trust advertisements.

"We don't have a choice on whether we *do* social media," it warns. "The question is how well we do it."

It turns out the video is a promotion for the creator Erik Qualman's book of the same title. While it makes a good point that social media can't be ignored, it's not that scary. In fact, social media is nothing more than a practice open house. It's just happening online.

Here are several guidelines from the book *Social Media is a Cocktail Party* by Jim Tobin and Lisa Braziel of Ignite Social Media:

- "The event goes on with or without you." Whether or not you are participating, people are talking about your practice online. Why not join the conversation?
- "Listen and mingle before you talk."
- "Different settings have different rules of etiquette." Just as you would behave differently at a children's birthday party than you would at a business networking lunch, Facebook requires a different decorum than LinkedIn. If Facebook is like an open house for the practice, then LinkedIn is the gathering of collaborating dentists.
- "You can ask for a little help from your friends." Once you build a base of followers who love you, they will write you stellar reviews and refer you more often. After all, anything for a friend.
- "Share information that doesn't benefit you." Apply the 80/20 rule here. Share 80% of the time about general social things that loosely reflect your practice's values, and 20% of the time hard facts about the practice.
- "Make it about them, not about you." People love to talk about themselves. Let them. When it's your turn, they will be all ears.

Let's dive deeper into best practices for Facebook. Post at least two to three times a week to stay visible. Anytime you get a comment on a post, comment back as soon as time permits to keep the conversation going. Make it possible for others to post on your page. (You can easily adjust this on your privacy settings.) Inviting others to post opens the door to your open house and invites others to be part of it. Have a personal *profile* on Facebook in addition to your business *page* to widen the circle of people whom you engage.

Finally, invite people to like your page. Message your friends on your personal profile first. Then include a "Like Us on Facebook" link in your email signature, on an iPad or tablet at your front desk, on your website – everywhere you can think of. Run a Facebook ad to get even more likes. We will explore Facebook ads in more depth in the next section, A System for Attracting Web Visitors.

Now for LinkedIn best practices. First and foremost, be sure to maintain a current profile. Potential patients and referrers will likely check you out online before calling, so you want them to see a complete and relevant profile. Don't make your profile a cut-and-paste of your curriculum vitae. Instead, draw readers in with elements from your Message and Design Equation.

Make your profile public by adjusting your settings. The more people who see you, the more new patients and referrals you will be exposed to.

Recommend others on LinkedIn. Don't just make endorsements by clicking on the buttons at the top of people's profiles. Take the time to write a short but detailed review about what they did for you and how it helped. Over time, many will do the same for you, and these reviews act as online referrals working for you. You can't beat word-of-mouth.

For even more exposure on LinkedIn, get involved in groups and discussion boards. Repurpose your blog postings to stay relevant and visible in multiple conversations. Anytime someone comments on something you post, be sure to comment back to keep the conversation going.

Let's talk about virality. That's virality, not to be confused with virility. Virality is the tendency to spread by word of mouth. It's all about cracking the code on getting noticed on social media.

Posts that get high virality, or are liked, commented on, and shared most often, are photos of the doctor and staff, babies or dogs (or better yet, babies with dogs), happy birthday posts (or better yet, happy wedding or happy new baby), and funny images or cartoons. Think: things that will make people smile and laugh.

Posts that get low virality include polls and questions that require too much thinking, and long posts that require too much reading. That's not as bad as it sounds. This is a social setting. No one likes the overt intellectual or long-winded talker to overtake the conversation. Keep it light.

It goes without saying to never post anything that may violate HIPAA regulations. But social media can be a slippery slope in this open-communications era. Train all the staff who are posting on social media to follow these guidelines:

1. If you wouldn't say it in an elevator, don't say it online.
2. Don't talk about patients, even in general terms.
3. Do talk about conditions, treatment, research.
4. Don't badmouth the competition, even subtly.
5. Do use humor carefully.
6. Keep personal posts on personal profiles and professional posts on professional pages.
7. When in doubt, leave it out.

(Source: http://www.kevinmd.com/blog/2011/06/7-tips-avoid-hipaa-violations-social-media.html)

Abe was right: It's impossible to please all of the people all of the time. Inevitably, you will get a negative social media post or comment. When it happens, behave just like you would in with a disgruntled patient acting out in your waiting room. Respond publicly to the original post. A simple, "Thank you for your feedback, we will do everything we can to rectify the situation" will do. Contact the patient personally. Be calm and understanding, listening intently until the patient has exhausted all emotion about the issue. If a resolution is reached, consider asking the patient to remove the post.

We all get the rare client who just can't be helped and doesn't want to behave rationally. As a last resort, use the setting that will ban the patient from posting.

Above all else, take the high road in social media. Behave with the ultimate decorum, and it will reflect favorably on you.

As always, remember that social media is only one tactic in your Balanced Marketing Formula. Avoid the temptation to get too carried away overinvesting time or thought to it. Use the *KABOOM!* method, and you will be able to stay the course for steady results.

A System for Attracting Web Visitors

The right tactics for attracting web visitors surface in nearly every dental practice's Balanced Marketing Formula. It's just a matter of figuring out which tactics are best to deploy at any given time. There are so many online tactics for attracting website visitors that even those who are marketing savvy can get overwhelmed.

As always, first consider the survey results. Would your existing patients search online for a practice like yours? Would they click on the ads, or only the organic search results? Would they follow you on Facebook? Cross off tactics from the list the data show that don't make as much sense for the practice.

Consider this funnel, the brainchild of Ryan Wilson of FiveFifty Digital Marketing, to further simplify the possibilities.

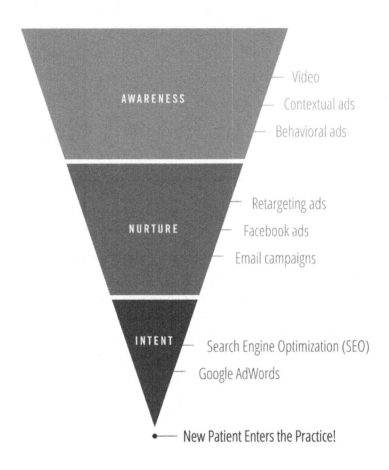

AWARENESS
— Video
— Contextual ads
— Behavioral ads

NURTURE
— Retargeting ads
— Facebook ads
— Email campaigns

INTENT
— Search Engine Optimization (SEO)
— Google AdWords

●— New Patient Enters the Practice!

Awareness

The top and largest section of Wilson's funnel is awareness. For new practices, the immediate goal is to increase awareness of the practice's offerings. No one knows about the practice yet, but they will soon with tactics of video, contextual ads, and behavioral ads.

Some dentists are under the false impression that they have to have video on their website in order to be highly visible by the search engines. While video might help, there are plenty of other more efficient tools to help with that exposure. Video production can be quite costly – $10,000 or more for a quality 3-minute spot – so tread lightly. A video makes most sense when it can be repurposed across several media. For example, a television spot can be added to the website homepage and shared across social media for maximum exposure.

Like retargeting ads, contextual and behavioral ads are colorfully designed, sometimes animated or flashy ads. Contextual ads appear on websites that have a context closely linked to your practice's offering. Behavioral ads appear on websites that match the online profile, or behavior, of those most likely to become patients.

All awareness tactics are typically best put into the hands of the experts. It's a big investment, but it can pay off big time.

In 2007 GoDaddy.com invested millions of dollars in Super Bowl ads that subsequently went viral online. While they didn't capture an immediate monetary return on investment, they reportedly drew 1.5 million visits to the GoDaddy.com website. Suddenly everyone knew GoDaddy.com.

This is top-of-mind awareness at its finest. After that game, whenever someone was ready to buy a website address, GoDaddy.com was the place to go.

Keep in mind that awareness can develop offline, too, with traditional marketing tactics like broadcast and billboard advertising. The most important thing is to do what's going to work best for your practice.

• • •

Nurture

Consider the next concept in Wilson's funnel: the pool of potential patients that you can nurture into the practice. These are patients who may have a need in the future, or who have lapsed in treatment but will need to return one day. While they are not ready to make an appointment today, they are likely to make an appointment in the next six months.

Nurture tactics help the practice show up in the right place at the right time. They most often include retargeting ads, Facebook ads, Facebook promoted posts, and email campaigns.

Retargeting ads include more than just text like Google AdWords. Often called banner ads, they are colorfully designed, sometimes animated or flashy ads that follow people around the web. Let's say a potential patient visits your website, but wanders off to a number of different sites. A banner ad for your practice can appear atop multiple pages on those other sites to keep your practice top-of-mind for the potential patient.

Facebook ads work in a similar manner, appearing in the newsfeeds of people who are likely to visit your practice one day. This visibility nurtures the potential patient to think of you when the time is right.

Facebook's "promoted" posts make it possible to plug the fact that certain patients like your practice page and may invite others to do the same. "This is a big deal," says Wilson, "because it's a referral for you working on your behalf with little or no effort from you."

What's more, daily posting on a practice Facebook page is the unpaid way to capture this mindshare and can be equally effective. As with SEO and Google AdWords, a one-two punch can pack the biggest bang.

Retargeting ads, Facebook ads and Facebook promoted posts are best handled by the experts.

Email campaigns are a great do-it-yourself option to nurture potential patients to take the next step. Push it beyond the typical practice newsletter. Create a series of emails that reflect your Message and Design Equation *and* have a clever twist. Consider repurposing your direct mail or print/billboard advertising campaigns into this digital medium for maximum effect.

• • •

Intent

Refer back to Wilson's funnel at the beginning of this section. The bottom and smallest area is packed full of people who seek a practice like yours. It's in every practice's best interest to make a concerted effort to reach the people who already have intent to see a doctor. "Right this very moment there are potential patients who already need your care," explains Wilson. "It's just a matter of scooping them up."

These are the folks who reside in the *intent* section of the funnel. They understand that they have a dental need, they know they have to seek out a dentist, and they are ready to make an appointment once they find the right dental practice. This is the low-hanging fruit. It's comparatively inexpensive to get intentional people to take that last step of calling for the appointment.

Intent tactics invite those people into the practice, and the tactics typically include Search engine optimization (SEO) and Google AdWords.

There's a big difference between SEO and AdWords:

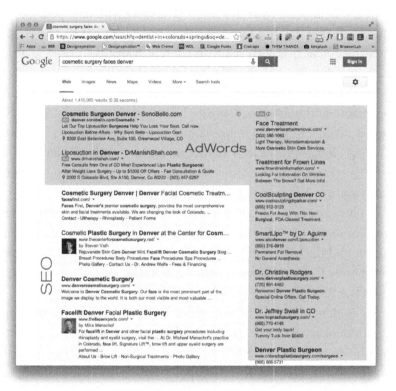

SEO drives websites to the top of the "organic" listings through methods of enriching website content. Google, Yahoo! and Bing crawl the web continuously to search out the most robust websites and present them as top choices for the keywords that are being searched. A search strategist will keep your name highly visible on those search engines by keeping your website healthy and active with relevant content, working links and a variety of other goodies that the search engines love.

SEO used to be a simple process of stuffing key words into a website and bolstering website headings with highly searched terms. Today it is a far more complex undertaking. On average, Google changes its search algorithm *every two days*. That means search strategists have to be continuously on the leading edge to keep your website on page one of the search results.

The more relevant the content and the more regular updates your website has, the more robust it appears to the search engines, and the higher it climbs in the search results. SEO for your website is like car maintenance – the tasks for upkeep continue over the lifetime of the vehicle.

Google AdWords is simply an online auction. Competing medical practices essentially outbid each other so their website ad shows most often. Each keyword, such as "Austin ophthalmologist," is given a dollar value, and the highest bidder's ad shows up first atop the page. The charge is triggered not when the ad shows but when someone clicks on the ad. Hence, the term pay-per-click advertising. This is where Google makes its money, by making it easy for small business owners to set up and manage their own campaigns.

Easy to set up and manage, sure. But it's more complicated to create a campaign that will *drive results*. A good search strategist will help select highly searched words and terms of a reasonable cost and that are most likely to covert clicks into paying patients. A good ad leads not to the website homepage but to a relevant landing page that echoes the offer in the ad. The landing page increases the likelihood that the potential patient will convert, or take the next step like call or make an appointment. Like any good ad, AdWords can get the customer in the door. The rest is up to you, which compels having a dynamic website.

It doesn't matter whether *you* are more apt to stick to the organic search results or to click on the ads on the Google results. It matters only how your potential patients behave online. Organic can help populate your website to page one of the search engines as a complement to AdWords.

SEO and Google AdWords are not do-it-yourself tactics. Lean on a strong search strategist to get the most out of your investment. A combination of both can drive patient traffic more quickly.

• • •

Each part of the funnel feeds into the next. Wilson advises, "If you have strong website traffic but people are not filling out the online form or calling in, that indicates the need to move people from nurture to intent. If your website traffic is low, that indicates a need for more awareness."

Some practices benefit from regularly running one or two tactics in each area of the funnel. Many simply stick to nurture tactics to maintain the status quo of patient traffic through top-of-mind awareness. All healthy practices keep coming back to the Balanced Marketing Formula to ensure a good spread of strategies, both online and offline.

"Eventually you will get to the point where you will have reached the number of people that you can affect," he explains. "Then you do more awareness to open up the funnel. Work from the bottom up.

"There's only so much you can do online," he continues. "No one will go online and book a $50,000 implant case, but there are other activities to optimize like 'Share your email address,' or 'Like us on Facebook.' Focus on those and move visitors down the funnel."

The great thing about online efforts is that they are highly measurable. Be sure to set up Google Analytics to track website traffic. Ask your agency for monthly reporting on your online marketing efforts. Consider these reports like you do your financial investment statements: look for overall trends but try not to get too caught up in the details.

With online promotion, so much of the decision happens before the patient even contacts the practice. Work the funnel with the guidelines provided here, and you will have applied the fruitful *KABOOM!* method to your online marketing, too!

Reputation Management Simplified

Reputation management is public relations happening on the web – it's all about keeping the practice's reputation squeaky clean online.

Specialists scour the web for the practice or doctor's name to uncover reviews and other content that may be damaging. Some reputation management services help cover up bad reviews by stuffing the web with good reviews or other content. This essentially pushes the less-than-stellar stuff off page one of the search engines. Reputation management can be incredibly time consuming and is best left to the experts – and only when absolutely necessary.

Consider first that it might not be necessary.

Ethically, reputation management can be challenging. After all, the First Amendment protects free speech, and reputation management tactics can be construed as censorship.

Reputation management can also backfire. One afternoon, a dentist friend called me in tears because a patient had written her a bad review. Why the long face? She had paid a service to correct it, and to bury the evidence they erected hundreds of dummy websites bearing her name, most with content that had nothing to do with her practice. The creation of these dummy websites is one way that reputation management services dilute the appearance of undesirable reviews on the search engines. These dummy websites were created not by a person but by an automated program, and inadvertently a few of the websites bore pornographic content. Had she done nothing, positive reviews would have filed in over time to offset the negative one. Instead, her reputation suffered. The correct remedy took years to take hold.

Be proactive rather than reactive. There are three things you can do today to boost your awareness of what's online about you. The more aware you are, the better positioned you are to immediately respond to any less-than-great reviews.

First, set up a Google Alert with the dentist's name and the practice name to receive regular updates about what is appearing on the web bearing your brand name.

Next, get social. The more active you are online, the more apt you are to get positive reviews and to see negative reviews, if any, as they happen.

Finally, add a patient communications service like Demand-Force, Lighthouse 360, or SolutionReach. For a reasonable fee, they help dental practices keep current patients engaged and happy with appointment reminders, digital check-in, email newsletters and opportunities to review the practice online. It's always easier to attract a positive review than it is to bury a negative one. What's more, these services are very easily managed by your front office staff.

What should you do if you get a bad review? As with social media, it's bound to happen at one time or another. The rule of thumb: Behave the same way you would if a patient voiced a negative opinion in your office. *Always respond.* To say nothing might exacerbate the issue by showing arrogance or ambivalence, implying agreement with the criticism. Type up a professional response and review it with another team member for objectivity and clarity before posting. Afterward, call the patient to hear his side of the story and offer a resolution. If all goes well, ask the patient to post his or her take on the resolution to the original online review. Even if they don't, your reply will show that you responded and did everything you could to take care of the patient.

By the way, an overall rating of four stars is great on a scale of five. Five-star reviews across the board suggest review stuffing, or "astroturfing," which undermines credibility.

Reputation is built every day in every way. When the practice is humming along at its best, it will be reflected online just as it is in offline circles. Be the best you can be, and glowing reviews will ensue. In this way, the *KABOOM!* method simplifies reputation management so you can focus on care.

Top 10 Mistakes in Online Promotion

1. **Believing slick salespeople.** There are no guarantees in online promotion. Walk away from anything that sounds too good to be true. "We will get you found on page one of Google tomorrow..."
2. **Same old site.** There are a lot of cookie-cutter templates out there, but you don't want to look like the dentist next door. At the same time, there's no need to hassle with an expensive custom website. A happy medium is a customizable WordPress theme. Pick a theme, and then add your own design to stand out.
3. **Dismemberment.** In your website, too, ditch the teeth-only photos in favor of full-face before-and-after shots. They tell a more compelling story to your potential patients.
4. **Bad shots.** Use crisp, clear images of the practice, dentist and staff in lieu of blurry or stock photos.
5. **Confusing navigation.** To keep the potential patient moving through the website and eventually to your door, narrow down the navigation to no more than seven pages or "rails" across the top and no more than five on each

dropdown. Group similar information on each page so the layout is digestible and well organized.

6. **Missing the opportunity.** Be sure the phone number, email address and links to the practice social media pages appear prominently on every webpage. Better yet, include a short form on every page with an engaging offer: "Share your email address and get our article, '10 Ways to Naturally Keep Teeth White and Bright.'"

7. **Missing the party.** People are talking about your practice online. Join the conversation. Join the social media revolution, with gusto.

8. **DIY on the cheap.** Attracting web visitors is to marketing as the all-on-four is to dentistry. (God forbid a layperson ever try that without his dentist!) Let go of the idea that a do-it-yourself solution will save money, and invest instead with an agency that can guide you through these tactics. It will pay off.

9. **Billboard at sea.** Your website is a billboard in the middle of the ocean until you make the effort to attract visitors. Start with an online marketing agency focused on intent tactics first (SEO and Google AdWords), since they are the easiest and least expensive way to attract people who already have the intention of finding a dentist like you.

10. **Reputation management run amok.** Instead of getting carried away worrying about bad reviews, focus on attracting great reviews by being your best.

PART FIVE

INTERNAL MARKETING

Internal marketing is the least expensive, most powerful and *most neglected* strategy.

What is internal marketing? It's a virtuous circle where happy employees cultivate happy patients, and happy patients bring more patients.

Practices often give special treatment to only *new* patients, to entice them to become patients, but not current ones who love them most.

Yet it's easier to retain current patients than it is to attract new ones. It's certainly more cost-effective to make your current patients happy and to inspire them to refer than it is to educate new people. A referred patient is likely to have a shorter learning curve and higher loyalty.

Current patients just show up! They might need a quick appointment reminder, but good patients just keep arriving. They also follow through with recommended treatment plans.

It's critical to *systemize* internal marketing in order to keep current patients coming back and referring.

There are two steps to implementing a healthy internal marketing strategy:

1. Inspire the team and patients to become avid fans of the practice.
2. Create systems for attracting referrals.

As it happens, internal marketing has little to do with external marketing tactics. It has more to do with motivated team members who have a high level of job satisfaction. To be successful, internal marketing takes team members who understand the practice vision, who are fiercely committed to reaching the practice goals, and who have tangible personal goals that are closely tied with the practice's growth. The team members are committed to delivering the same high level of service and quality in every patient interaction.

Notice that the team comes before the patients. Again, happy team equals happy patients. You can't have the latter without the former.

A few external marketing tactics do cross over to internal marketing. These tactics touch current patients and inspire them to remain loyal and to refer their friends. Examples include patient newsletters, formally presented treatment plans, open houses, referral cards, in-office promotional materials, social media interaction, and appointment reminders. Even the new patient intake process is a form of internal marketing communication. The way each of these tactics is handled should tie back to the practice's vision, goals, and the Message and Design Equation and Balanced Marketing Formula.

The nuances of internal marketing are endless. *How the phone is answered. Whether shirts are tucked in. What it says about the practice when the doctor runs late.* The patient surveys will reveal what's appealing to team members and patients, and what's not. Look back for what your team shared in the surveys about the practice, which can easily springboard into the creation of mission, vision and values.

The mission answers the question, What is the practice's main purpose today? It's why you and your team show up to work every day. It's very likely tied to your Message and Design Equation.

The vision answers the question, What is the practice's ideal future? You might start your vision statement with the phrase, "To create a world where..."

The values answer the question, What is the practice's core ideology? Here's an example of a values statement:

We value...

o **Choice** – Our dentists and supporting team guide patients in making the best possible choices for their dental health. We provide patients with a choice of treatment options that will best fit their needs, schedule and budget.

o **Philanthropy** – We give back to the community in our everyday work and far beyond. We believe that giving is receiving.

o **Collaboration** – We partner with other dentists and healthcare professionals to provide the best possible care for all patients. We inspire our team to communicate with each other on a regular basis in order to optimize care. And we encourage patients to join the conversation for the best possible outcome.

Internal marketing circles back to brand. It's all about perception and *experience*. When you make a patient a promise, verbally or non-verbally, and you deliver on that promise, your patient has an excellent experience. Patients who have an excellent experience keep coming back, and they keep like-minded patients crossing your threshold.

Share the practice goal, mission, vision and values with your team. Inspire them to get on board, and watch them sail the ship.

Systemize your team's delivery of excellence. It's a spectacular thing when it all comes together – and it's even easier with the *KABOOM!* method.

CHECKLIST FOR TEAM TRAINING

Internal marketing begins on the inside. Think of the practice goal, mission, vision and values as the internal marketing *core*. Once the core is established, share it with the team. Next, involve them over the course of several weeks in recalibrating all areas of the practice to match the core:

✓ *Monitor how the phone is answered.* What is the voice that your new patients hear? What phrases and words do the receptionists use, and how do they align with the practice's core? Is the way the phone is answered congruent with your core?

✓ *Take inventory of what the team is wearing.* Is that wardrobe a reflection of your core? Or does it need updating?

✓ *Review patient intake forms.* Are they branded with your logo and colors? Are they easy to fill out? Are they online or on paper, and which do your patients prefer? Do you walk patients through the forms, or just leave forms with the patient? What fits best with your core?

✓ *Take a walk through office.* Do the décor and wall hangings reflect your vision and demonstrate credibility? Does it feel warm and friendly, or cold and clinical? How can the office be updated to better match your core?

✓ *Review the flow of your initial consultation.* Is it calming and welcoming? What words and phrases do you often use? Are the terms you use understandable, or too clinical for the patient? What is your tactic for "closing the deal," or getting the patient to sign on for treatment? How can you make it easier for patients to know and trust you and thereby consent to your treatment plan? How does the initial consultation communicate your core?

✓ *Observe how the patient flows through the practice.* Is the experience similar with each interaction – front desk staff to doctor to assistant or hygienist? Where is additional training needed to get everyone in lockstep on delivering excellent patient care that's in keeping with your core?

✓ *Collect patient correspondence and consider it in full.* Is your correspondence a reflection of your core, or just a set of cookie-cutter templates? How can you make your correspondence unique to your core? How can you go overboard to please the patient so he or she will remain loyal to you and refer to you more often?

"The aim is to create raving fans inside the practice," explains Kim McGuire of Fortune Management. "Start from the inside to create a wow experience." In McGuire's world, this level of excellence extends beyond well-running systems. That's certainly part of the equation, but it's just as important that team members are in sync with the practice core.

"You can ask for referrals," says McGuire, "but if team commitment is broken on the inside then the referral strategy is never going to stick."

She goes on to explain, "One of the big things that you always start with is team members' belief systems around asking for referrals. Some people think of it as begging or a sign of desperation. The reality is, if you offer amazing care that you believe in, then you know that all of your friends, family and circles beyond deserve that level of care. And that belief makes it easier to ask for the referral."

Start with the team, and the practice referral strategy will yield strong results. As with everything else in the *KABOOM!* method, team training is just one part of the overall strategy. Let's look next at a system for attracting more referrals.

REFERRAL MINING ON LINKEDIN

Dentists can certainly reach out to other dentists to introduce themselves and invite referrals. State-level associations, local organizations and study clubs are an extension of this process, but they require membership fees and time-consuming face time. It is no doubt important to include these tactics in a referral strategy. Additionally, it's critical to add the online version of networking.

Referral mining on LinkedIn is the process of hosting an online open house to meet and greet people who may bring patients into the practice. This tactic is particularly fruitful for specialty practices and for dentists who rely heavily on referrals for new patient traffic. It's a great way to exponentially expand your network of referrers relatively quickly.

The patient surveys will reveal if this is best for you. If so, start by completing your LinkedIn profile, as detailed in Demystifying Social Media in Part Four.

Then it's time to invite people to your open house and build your network. Here's how:

1. *Search.* In the search box at the top of LinkedIn, type in the names of industry friends and current referrers –

both dentists and referrers who are not dentists. Think of anyone who you would invite to an open house, anyone whose email address you have. Connect first with everyone you already know. Click "Connect," and if prompted, enter their email address.

2. *Branch Out.* On the upper right corner of your LinkedIn home page, click on "People You May Know." This will produce a list of more people that you can connect with. Scroll down the page and click "Connect" next to anyone you would like to know better. An invitation will be sent to them. Watch carefully for acceptances.

3. *Invite more people.* Make it a weekly routine to connect with more people from "People You May Know." An invitation will be sent to them. Now sit back and watch as they accept your invitation and your online open house comes to life.

LinkedIn changes the rules from time to time, but the basics stay the same: connect with your friends, connect with their friends, and once connected, start a friendly conversation.

Once a new connection accepts your request, send them a friendly private message. The email that you received notifying you of their acceptance will have a button that says "Send a Message" – simply click there and follow the prompts. Keep the email short, conversational and friendly, three to five sentences max. Ask for a lunch meeting or phone call, and propose a date and time.

When you connect offline, share your practice core and ask about theirs. Explore how best to work together. Focus first on how you can help them, and next on how they might help you.

Next, sort through the details of how to make referring easy for them. The simpler the process, the more apt they are to send you new patients.

And the more often they send you new patients, the more stable the practice becomes. Just another gift from the *KABOOM!* method.

Referral System

Inevitably, referrals trickle in from time to time by virtue of your reputation. The trick to growing word-of-mouth is to systemize the process of attracting referrals for steady new patient flow. As often as possible, be best to those who love you most and they will become raving fans of the practice and more steadily send new patients your way. There are three parts to this system: List, Ask, Remind.

List

Make a list of those you know who are most likely to refer to the practice. Include the names of current patients and dentists or other healthcare practitioners who tend to refer. Then cast a wider net, jotting down the names of people who you believe *would* refer if they were prompted.

Once a week, make it a point to connect in a meaningful way with each person on the list. Small gestures go a long way. Comment about a post on a referring patient's personal Facebook page. Send a referring dentist a book, an article, a funny video or something else of interest. Take a referring practitioner out for coffee or lunch. Send a referring practice a basket of fruit to thank them. Take patients or dentists who refer most often to a local sporting event. These tactics keep you top-of-mind, which is the heart of marketing.

Next, consider running a referral contest. People are like toddlers in that they're willing to do just about anything for a small prize. Align the reward with your Message and Design Equation. For example, my friend Dr. Kearney learned on his surveys that he's best known for his sense of adventure, coupled with his straightforward care. He ran a referral contest reflecting that. Patients who made a word-of-mouth recommendation over a three-month-period were entered to win a hot-air balloon ride with Adventures Out West.

After the referral comes in, reward referrers with a $5 gift card to a coffee shop or other low-cost diversion that is in keeping with your practice's Message and Design Equation. Mail a handwritten thank-you note to anyone who refers. Ask the referrer how *you* can help *them*, and deliver on their request. The most valuable appreciation you can give is to connect a referrer with other people who can exponentially help them.

The list reminds you to subtly remind others to send new patients your way. What's next is the art of the Ask.

• • •

Ask

McGuire reminds us, "You have to actually ask people for referrals. The moment that you connect with people is the time to ask. Directly after the patient gives you or the practice a compliment, ask 'Would you please refer our practice?' Or prompt a compliment: 'How was your experience today? What would have made it outstanding? Would you consider referring friends and family our way?'"

Make it natural. Train yourself and the team to be alert to those moments of genuine connection, and to casually yet clearly frame the question. Role-play in team meetings so it becomes a comfortable communication for everyone. McGuire suggests saying something like, "We love patients like you. We would love to see your friends and family. Would you be able to refer us?"

The Ask is more effective coming from a team member than the dentist. "It's not their name on the door," explains McGuire, "So it feels much softer." This approach also preserves the dentist's integrity as a clinical expert rather than a business development promoter.

Then again, some doctors are naturals at the Ask. Follow your gut. "It's a refined skill," McGuire adds. "Practice makes perfect."

• • •

Remind

Put something in patients' hands that reminds them to refer. At the end of each appointment, offer the patient a few referral cards. These can be simple business cards that have a fill-in-the-blanks for patient name and read, "John Smith referred me as a new patient. As a reward, we will both receive $25 towards any service." The patient willingly hands them out to their friends and family, and the practice attracts new patients.

Avoid offering discounts to new patient leads that originate from direct mail or website attraction tactics. But feel free to use incentives with current and referred patients, since they are the highest value customers.

Align your reminder cards and offer with your Message and Design Equation. Meet with your team to decide how many cards to give out each day and which patients should receive them. Timing matters. If a patient seems especially happy after the visit, share the card.

Another way to remind is with a professional presentation to share with potential referring dentists and healthcare practitioners. A simple PowerPoint will suffice to showcase professional credentials and success stories. The presentation should also convey the process for integrating referred patients into your practice, and your strategy for communicating care back to the referring doctor. Consider leaving several referral forms with doctors, reminding them to refer and making it easy for them to send a patient.

The beauty of referral cards and forms is that they retain some shelf life. When patients carry your cards in their wallets or doctors store your referral forms in their front office, they will be reminded over and over again to refer to you.

• • •

Once the team gets used to the referral system, it won't have to be so formal or structured. Asking people will become second nature.

If you see patient traffic leveling out or dropping off, that's the time to reexamine your referral system. Recalibrating this system is the easiest, cheapest way to jumpstart business. Resist the temptation to spend time and money attracting new patients from other sources first. The referred patient enters the practice more easily, is more likely to accept treatment, and is more likely to become a lifetime patient and an avid fan of the practice. Talk about tapping the *KABOOM!* method!

THE TRIFECTA

Internal functions are integral to making your marketing strategy work. This is the trifecta of internal functions: leadership, systems/processes, and cash flow. The trifecta is the foundational support to your marketing, like a tripod for a camera. When any leg of the trifecta is out of whack, your marketing is less effective.

Leadership

Warren Bennis says, "Leadership is the capacity to translate vision into reality."

By that definition, anyone in the practice can be a leader, but leadership starts at the top. The dentist must be clear about the vision, overall goal, and goals for marketing. He or she must find a way to clearly and regularly communicate this knowledge to the team. The dentist must *inspire* the team.

Leadership transcends one powerful person leading the group. True leadership begins when every team member becomes a leader. A team of leaders has a shared practice vision and a passion for the common goal. Each develops ideas, processes and systems for reaching the practice goal.

Leaders are also hungry to reach their personal goals. They understand how the practice can help them fulfill those wishes and dreams.

Leaders are thinkers, not doers. They come to you with solutions not problems. Each is indispensable to the function of the practice. They are insatiably positive; they avoid gossip and negativity. They are aware of what propels the practice forward, always alert to pitfalls that might hurt the practice.

Leaders possess a deep-rooted self-respect and therefore are able to extend genuine respect to everything and everyone around them. They lift others up. Leaders are natural caregivers.

When everyone in the practice is a leader, everyone is empowered to execute the marketing to propel the practice in the right direction.

The opposites of these traits in any team member indicate that there is room for leadership improvement. Anytime there is a hole in leadership, the marketing (and other systems) will suffer. Inspire your team to become the best leaders that they can be. Those who aren't able to meet the challenge will eventually exit the practice. The remaining team will retain the power to take the practice to the next level.

The best professional to help with this transition is a practice coach, not to be confused with a practice management consultant. The coach focuses on improving *people* while the consultant works on improving *systems*. That brings us to the second leg in the trifecta...

• • •

Systems/Processes

Internal systems and processes allow the practice to work for you, freeing you up to focus on care. Are you still running payroll?

Is anyone else empowered with hiring decisions? Are you the sole person in charge of marketing?

Setting up internal structures to automate these functions and outsource certain functions to the experts will simplify business operations and get you back to what you do best.

Some necessary systems are obvious: filing, phone, billing and bookkeeping, patient database. Other systems are more nuanced: a method for purchasing supplies and equipment, a plan for upkeep of the facility and premises, a system for streamlining work with vendors.

Here are just a few processes that are often missing: a process for scheduling appointments, for patient intake, for intuitively storing patient forms and information, for orienting new team members, for integrating associates. When processes are missing, these functions feel arduous.

Excellent systems and processes address the question, "What is the most efficient way of doing this?"

When systems and processes are lacking, the effectiveness of the marketing suffers. Marketing leads the horse to water, and systems and processes make it drink. For example, a robust marketing strategy might attract new patients to the practice. When that new patient calls in, the phones must work properly, the intake process must be seamless, the billing process buttoned up, the follow-up process dialed, etc. When the systems and processes work in synergy, the patient has an excellent overall experience, which inspires him or her to remain loyal to the practice and bring more new patients into the practice.

To thoroughly audit your systems and processes, The Medical Group Management Association advises examining key areas of the practice:

- Business operations
- Financial management
- Human resources management
- Information management
- Organizational governance
- Patient care systems
- Quality management
- Risk management

(Source: http://www.cmgma.org/site/body-of-knowledge.htm?)
As the practice grows, old systems break down and new systems replace them. A good practice management consultant can help guide this as an ongoing process.

• • •

Cash Flow

A cash flow solution is distinct from bookkeeping or accounting, which reflect historical views on the practice finances. The term cash flow refers to the money that will come in and go out of the practice in the next few weeks and months. It is a forward-looking view on the finances, a forecast. The process of projecting cash flow is sometimes called revenue cycle management.

A good eye on cash flow allows you to hire staff, purchase equipment, invest in marketing and otherwise expand with confidence. Strong cash flow gives insight on what works. For example, you can fully consider projected expenses and returns in preparation for launching a newly minted Balance Marketing Formula. In this way, the cash flow forecasting process helps further ground the marketing in strategy rather than guesswork.

A cash flow consultant can provide accurate projections for the next six to twelve months. The cash flow report typically shows for each week or each month how much money is in the bank, what patient fees are projected to be collected, what expenses and liabilities are anticipated and what profit is expected. If the practice is experiencing weak cash flow, a week-by-week projection can provide granular data to get back on the right track. If cash flow is moderate to strong, a month-by-month projection is all the information you need.

Cash flow is fuel that propels the marketing machine. When cash flow is weak, it seems impossible to invest regularly in marketing that will maintain steady patient flow and strong production. When cash flow is strong and marketing becomes a standard monthly investment, marketing efforts are consistent and results are, too.

• • •

The practice with excellent leadership, systems/processes, and cash flow benefits the most from the *KABOOM!* method. Strengthen each leg in your trifecta for the ultimate in practice stability.

Top 10 Mistakes in Internal Marketing

1. **Neglect.** When patient traffic drops off, very few dentists think to ratchet up internal marketing *first*. In fact, most of them forget internal marketing altogether. The opposite of "neglect" is "respect." When you focus on internal marketing you focus on respect – for the team, the patients, and the referrers.

2. **Cart Before the Horse.** Don't put patients before the team, or new patients before existing ones. Be sure to nurture the team first, then current patients, then new patients. Though it may seem counterintuitive, this priority level will position you to *always* be attracting a steady flow of patients and production.

3. **Training instead of inspiring.** Your team is your most valuable asset. Go beyond teaching them. Excite them!

4. **Going it alone.** Every aspect of internal marketing is meant to be deployed as a *team*, not by you alone. Go beyond becoming a great leader yourself. Empower each of your teammates to become leaders.

5. **Failing to ask.** You must actually solicit referrals. It's a small but critical step in the process of attracting

referrals, and believe it or not it's often forgotten. If you want people to take action, tell them specifically what you want them to do.

6. **Overkill.** Avoid over-asking for referrals, which can offend people. Wait until a connection is made and the time feels right. You will know when.

7. **Doing business apologetically.** What you do as a dentist transforms lives. Own it. Go out and boldly ask for referrals.

8. **Stopping short.** Sure, you can bump into potential referring patients and doctors out in the community. But your efforts will take less time and produce more results if you actively seek out referrals on LinkedIn, too.

9. **Waiting.** Rather than waiting for referrals to trickle in spontaneously, systemize the process of attracting them to grow the practice.

10. **Staggering.** If any leg of your tripod is broken, the camera won't work well. Be sure that your leadership, practice systems and processes, and cash flow are strong to support your marketing efforts.

Afterword

We have entered an Age of Fear in dentistry. Fear that the Affordable Care Act will be our demise. Fear of the trending consolidation of providers. Fear of corporate dentistry. Fear of encroaching competitors. Fear of the daunting shift to digital records. Fear of the shift to digital marketing.

The word "science," is Latin for "knowledge." Ralph Waldo Emerson said, "Knowledge is the antidote for fear."

The more knowledge you have about marketing, the more able you are to find a cure for these fears. You will benefit from a cure that allows you to attract the right kind of patients and to thrive in solo or small practice. You can stand out in even the most saturated markets.

And more than all of that, you can concentrate on changing the things that will make your profession easier, more fruitful and more rewarding. Thanks to the *KABOOM!* method to simplify the process of getting explosive marketing results, you can finally focus on what matters most: care.

EXERCISE #1

YOUR MESSAGE AND DESIGN EQUATION

Use this exercise to formulate your practice's Message and Design Equation. Download a larger copy of this exercise at www.bigbuzzinc.com/kaboom.

1. What are three ways that my patients say my practice is different and better than other practices? (Be sure that these are benefits, not features. Gentle care is a benefit. Sedation is a feature. Lastly, each should be objective and, where possible, quantifiable. Think, "Patients are warmly greeted by three staff members before entering the operatory," as opposed to, "Patients think we're nice.")

   ○ _____

   ○ _____

   ○ _____

2. What is the No. 1 thing people like best about the practice? (It's usually the benefit that comes up over and over again in survey responses. If you keep seeing "funny," "laughter," and "smiling" in the survey responses, the No. 1 thing may be "humor." And remember, more often than not patients are drawn in by *non-clinical* benefits. They are buying a relationship with you, not just your dental expertise.)

Message: _____

Design:
(Describe below, in writing or as a collage of pictures, the types of imagery, illustration, photography, etc. that best represent your message.)

YOUR BALANCED MARKETING FORMULA

Use this exercise to formulate your practice's Balanced Marketing Formula. Download a larger copy of this exercise at www.bigbuzzinc.com/kaboom.

SAMPLE BALANCED MARKETING FORMULA

Use this sample to guide you in formulating your practice's Balanced Marketing Formula. Download a larger copy of this sample at www. bigbuzzinc.com/kaboom.

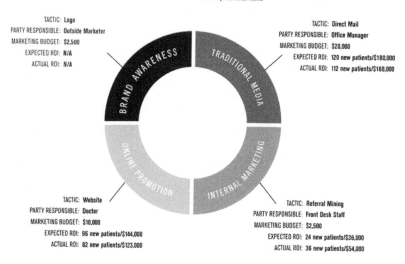

TOTAL ANNUAL MARKETING BUDGET: $35,000
AVERAGE PATIENT VALUE: $1,500
TOTAL ANNUAL EXPECTED ROI: 240 new patients/$360,000
TOTAL ACTUAL ROI: 230 new patients/$345,000

TACTIC: Logo
PARTY RESPONSIBLE: Outside Marketer
MARKETING BUDGET: $2,500
EXPECTED ROI: N/A
ACTUAL ROI: N/A

TACTIC: Direct Mail
PARTY RESPONSIBLE: Office Manager
MARKETING BUDGET: $20,000
EXPECTED ROI: 120 new patients/$180,000
ACTUAL ROI: 112 new patients/$168,000

TACTIC: Website
PARTY RESPONSIBLE: Doctor
MARKETING BUDGET: $10,000
EXPECTED ROI: 96 new patients/$144,000
ACTUAL ROI: 82 new patients/$123,000

TACTIC: Referral Mining
PARTY RESPONSIBLE: Front Desk Staff
MARKETING BUDGET: $2,500
EXPECTED ROI: 24 new patients/$36,000
ACTUAL ROI: 36 new patients/$54,000

BRAND AWARENESS
TRADITIONAL MEDIA
ONLINE PROMOTION
INTERNAL MARKETING

Stay On The Cutting Edge

Like what you read and want more? Here are two easy ways that you can receive timely and relevant content updates that build upon the *KABOOM!* method and that guide the overall business side of your dental practice:

1. Go to www.bigbuzzinc.com, enter your email address to receive regular content updates via email.
2. Like us on Facebook at www.facebook.com/BigBuzz-Brands to get regular content updates in your newsfeed.

Get more thought-provoking insights directly from Wendy O'Donovan Phillips with no additional cost to you. All content is crafted exclusively by Wendy for the purpose of inspiring change and growth in your practice.

ACKNOWLEDGEMENTS

Many people helped make this book, beginning with my mom, Bonnie O'Donovan, who has been my staunch supporter throughout my life and career. Too, she demonstrated excellence in healthcare to me, having worked for four decades in the industry. My dad, Bill O'Donovan, edited this book. To quote Mary Baker Eddy, he was at once "wise and gentle and strong and fearless" in his editing. He is the reason I am in communications; having spent four decades in the newspaper industry, he has instilled in me a love for the written word and a passion for the art of persuasion.

My husband, Trevor Lee Phillips has always stood by me and cheered me on, even when my marketing agency and this book were mere pipe dreams. I get to check "write a book" off my bucket list thanks to his advocacy. I am grateful to him also for caring for our daughter, Willa, late at night and on weekends while I wrote.

My team members at work are the best leaders I know: Molly Watkins, Andrew Zareck, Randall Hartman, Katie Weingardt, Shannon Dils, and Christy Kruzick. Molly project managed the book. Randall contributed the referral mining on LinkedIn idea.

Andrew contributed the foundation for the section on logos, and he created all of the art for the book. Katie and Christy proofed the manuscript. They all impeccably held down the agency while I was writing. Alicia Marie provided the coaching that has led me here and the inspiration for the section on leadership. Brenda Abdilla kept me calm, and along with Dr. Brett Kessler and Mary LoVerde provided mentorship and manuscript feedback. Many professionals let me learn from their example: Dr. Brandon Hall, Dr. Christopher Cote, Dr. Nicolette Picerno, Dr. Chris Roberts, Dr. Dianne Stone, Dr. Jim Kearney, Drs. David and Stuart Bennett, Dr. Thomas Jennings, Dr. Jennifer Rankin, Dr. Michael Mingle, and the late Dr. David Winn. Debra Robinson and Kim Eickhoff taught me to appreciate cash flow and financial processes. Lisa Stemmer, Shayne Harris, Ryan Wilson and Kim McGuire provided insights and contributions. Mark Weaver provided the means for me to finish the last mile of this marathon.

I'm lucky to have each one of you in my corner.